GASTRIC SLEEVE COOKBOOK 2024

Easy delicious meal plans including health benefits to eat well and keep the weight off with nutritional values

MARY N. MAXWELL

Introduction..**5**

Understanding Gastric Sleeve Surgery... 5

Preparing for Success: Pre- and Post-Surgical Guidelines............................. 6

Importance of Nutrition Following Surgery... 8

Psychological Preparation... 8

Managing Expectations... 9

CHAPTER 1..**11**

Essential Kitchen Tools and Ingredients... 11

Essential Kitchen Tools for Gastric Sleeve Patients...................................... 11

Key Ingredients for Healthier Cooking.. 12

CHAPTER 2..**17**

Breakfasts for Champions...17

CHAPTER 3..**27**

Satisfying Soups and Salads.. 27

Tips for Creating Balanced and Filling Soups and Salads.............................33

Deliciously Lean Protein Dishes:.. 36

CHAPTER 4..**47**

Veggie-Centric Creations:..47

CHAPTER 5..**58**

Smart Snacks and Small Bites:.. 58

CHAPTER 6..**64**

Delectable Desserts.. 64

CHAPTER 7..**69**

Hydration and Beverage...69

CHAPTER 8..**74**

Meal Planning and Preparation Strategies..74

Weekly Meal Planning Guidelines..74

Tips for Batch Cooking and Freezing... 75

Dining Out Strategies for Success...77

Maintaining Motivation and Lifestyle Changes... 79

Setting Realistic Goals... 79

Overcoming Challenges and Plateaus..80

Celebrating Successes Along the Way..82

CHAPTER 9..**85**

Resources and Support..85

Support Groups and Communities..85

Additional Tips and Advice for Long-Term Success..87

30 DAYS MEAL PLAN..**91**

INTRODUCTION

Gastric sleeve surgery, also known as sleeve gastrectomy, is a surgical technique that removes a large section of the stomach to produce a smaller, sleeve-shaped pouch. This surgery is widely used to treat extreme obesity, especially when other weight loss procedures have been unsuccessful.

Understanding Gastric Sleeve Surgery.

Gastric sleeve surgery works by lowering the size of the stomach, limiting the amount of food that may be eaten at once. During the treatment, the physician eliminates 75-80% of the stomach, leaving behind a small tube or sleeve-shaped stomach pouch. This smaller stomach pouch stores substantially less food than the original stomach, resulting in feelings of fullness and pleasure with lower meals.

Laparoscopic surgery is often conducted through tiny incisions using a camera-equipped surgical equipment known as a laparoscope. This minimally invasive procedure provides for speedier recovery, less discomfort, and a decreased chance of problems than standard open surgery.

One of the primary benefits of gastric sleeve surgery is that it does not entail rerouting or bypassing the intestines, as other weight loss operations do. This implies that vitamin absorption is mostly unchanged, lowering the danger of nutritional deficiencies.

Following surgery, the remaining section of the stomach continues to operate properly, generating digestive fluids and enzymes that help in digesting. However, the smaller stomach capacity reduces the amount of food that can be ingested, resulting in lower calorie intake and, eventually, weight reduction.

Preparing for Success: Pre- and Post-Surgical Guidelines

Preparation for gastric sleeve surgery begins well before the operation. Patients are thoroughly medically examined to determine that they are suitable candidates for surgery. This evaluation usually includes an assessment of overall health, nutritional status, psychological well-being, and readiness for lifestyle changes.

Prior to surgery, patients may be needed to adhere to a pre-operative diet in order to shrink the liver and limit the chance of problems. This diet often includes high-protein, low-carbohydrate, and low-calorie meals, as well as lots of fluids. Patients may also be urged to stop smoking and avoid certain drugs that raise the risk of bleeding or other problems.

Patients require a time of recuperation and adjustment after surgery to allow their bodies to adapt to the alterations caused by the treatment. Post-operative instructions usually include:

1. Dietary Guidelines: Patients begin on a liquid diet, then proceed to pureed meals, soft foods, and, finally, solid foods over many weeks. To avoid issues and enhance recovery, strictly adhere to the specified eating plan.

2. Physical Activity: While severe exercise is often avoided in the early post-operative period, patients are urged to participate in modest physical activity, such as walking, to improve circulation, prevent blood clots, and assist in recuperation.

3. Medication Management: Patients may be offered pain relievers and/or antibiotics to alleviate discomfort and lower the risk of infection. It is essential to take drugs as prescribed by the healthcare practitioner.

4. Follow-Up Care: Regular follow-up meetings with the surgical team are critical for monitoring progress, addressing any concerns or issues, and providing continuous support and advice.

5. Lifestyle adjustments: Gastric sleeve surgery is not a fast answer for weight reduction, but rather a tool to help patients make lifestyle adjustments. To ensure long-term success, patients are advised to establish good eating habits, engage in regular physical activity, and make durable lifestyle changes.

Importance of Nutrition Following Surgery

Nutrition is critical to the effectiveness of gastric sleeve surgery and the general health and well-being of patients. Following surgery, the lower stomach capacity and changes in digestion necessitate careful consideration of food choices to maintain appropriate nutrition while supporting weight reduction.

The key concepts of diet following gastric sleeve surgery are:

1. Protein Intake: Protein is required for healing, muscle regeneration, and maintaining lean body mass. Patients are recommended to eat protein-rich meals at every meal to satisfy their dietary requirements. Lean protein sources include poultry, fish, eggs, tofu, lentils, and low-fat dairy products.

2. Hydration: Adequate hydration is vital for good health and digestion. Patients should attempt to consume enough fluids throughout the day, emphasizingFurthermore, it is critical to understand that gastric sleeve surgery is not a one-size-fits-all treatment. Each patient's path is unique, and personalized treatment and support are critical to long-term success. The decision to have gastric sleeve surgery should be made after consulting with a multidisciplinary team of healthcare professionals, including bariatric surgeons, registered dietitians, psychologists, and other specialists who can provide comprehensive pre- and post-operative care.

Psychological Preparation

In addition to physical preparation, patients must be intellectually and emotionally prepared for the challenges and adjustments associated with gastric sleeve surgery. Many people suffering from extreme obesity have a lengthy history of unsuccessful weight loss attempts, societal shame, and emotional discomfort. As a result, addressing psychological issues before and after surgery is critical.

Pre-surgery psychological examinations are frequently used to examine patients' mental health, motivation, and preparation for surgery. This examination may include a screening for eating disorders, depression, anxiety, and other psychological conditions that might affect surgical results. Patients may also receive counseling or join support groups to address emotional problems and learn coping methods for life after surgery.

Patients may feel a variety of emotions following surgery, including exhilaration, worry, and frustration as they deal with the physical and emotional changes that come with weight reduction. It is critical that patients have access to continuing support and tools to help them adjust to their new lifestyle and deal with any issues that may emerge.

Managing Expectations

While gastric sleeve surgery can change people's lives, it's important to have realistic expectations about the procedure's outcomes and limitations. Weight reduction outcomes differ from person to person and are impacted by variables such as age, beginning weight, overall health, commitment to food and lifestyle modifications, and support network.

Patients should understand that gastric sleeve surgery can help them lose weight and improve their health, but it is not a cure-all for obesity. Long-term success necessitates a commitment to lifetime diet, exercise, and behavior adjustments. While considerable weight reduction can be accomplished in the months following surgery, individuals may have weight swings over time and may not meet their long-term weight loss objectives immediately.

It is also vital to understand that gastric sleeve surgery carries risks and problems. Infection, hemorrhage, blood clots, leaks at the surgery site, and nutritional deficits are all possible consequences, albeit they are uncommon. Patients should be properly educated about the risks and advantages of surgery, as well as having reasonable expectations for the recovery process and possible results.

In conclusion, gastric sleeve surgery is an effective tool for people suffering from extreme obesity, providing a road to considerable weight loss and improved health outcomes. Understanding the surgical technique, planning for success with pre- and post-operative instructions, addressing psychological variables, regulating expectations, and committing to lifestyle changes are all critical stages toward long-term success.

Patients who work closely with a multidisciplinary team of healthcare specialists, adopt good lifestyle choices, and seek continuous support and resources can optimize the advantages of gastric sleeve surgery and live a happier, more satisfying life. While the path might be difficult at times, the benefits of better health, more energy, and a higher quality of life make it all worthwhile.

CHAPTER 1

Essential Kitchen Tools and Ingredients

Cooking and preparing meals at home can be critical to success after gastric sleeve surgery. Having the correct kitchen tools and supplies on hand may help you prepare meals more easily, efficiently, and enjoyably. In this complete guide, we'll look at essential kitchen tools and ingredients for gastric sleeve patients, allowing you to prepare tasty, healthy meals that support your health and weight reduction objectives.

Essential Kitchen Tools for Gastric Sleeve Patients

1. Food Scale: A food scale is an essential tool for portion management and precise measuring of materials. Gastric sleeve patients must be cautious of meal sizes to avoid overeating and ensuring they obtain enough nutrition.

2. Measuring Cups and Spoons: Measuring cups and spoons are required for correct measurement of substances, especially when following recipes. This helps to maintain consistency in portion sizes and calorie consumption.

3. Sharp Chef's Knife: A sharp chef's knife makes it easier and safer to chop, dice, and slice fruits, vegetables, and meats. Investing in a high-quality knife can help you prepare meals faster and enjoy cooking more.

4. Cutting Board: A sturdy cutting board offers a steady platform for slicing and prepping food. Look for a cutting board made of a nonporous material, such as plastic or bamboo, that is simple to clean and disinfect.

5. Blender or Food Processor: A blender or food processor is extremely useful for making

smoothies, purees, sauces, and soups. These devices can assist gastric sleeve patients integrate a range of nutrient-dense meals into their diet in a practical and tasty manner.

6. Non-Stick Cookware: Non-stick cookware simplifies cooking with less oil or grease and lowers the likelihood of food sticking to the pan. Choose high-quality nonstick cookware and pots that are PFOA-free and dishwasher safe for easy cleanup.

7. Steamer Basket: A steamer basket is a great way to prepare vegetables, fish, and cereals while retaining their natural taste, color, and nutrients. Steaming is a healthy cooking method that uses less extra fat and helps to preserve the nutritional value of foods.

8. Silicone Baking Mats: Silicone baking mats provide a nonstick surface for baking, eliminating the need for grease or parchment paper. They're great for making low-fat, high-protein desserts like protein bars, muffins, and cookies.

9. Herb & Spice Grinder: Freshly ground herbs and spices may enhance the flavor of foods without adding unnecessary calories or sodium. Investing in a high-quality herb and spice grinder enables gastric sleeve patients to enjoy tasty, aromatic meals while reducing the need for extra salt and fat.

10. Storage Containers: Having a choice of storage containers in different sizes makes it simple to divide out meals, store leftovers, and plan meals for the week ahead. To maximize adaptability, look for BPA-free containers that may be used in the microwave, dishwasher, and freezer.

By stocking your kitchen with these basic items, you'll be ready to cook nutritious, tasty meals that will help you lose weight and improve your overall health following gastric sleeve surgery.

Key Ingredients for Healthier Cooking

1. Lean Proteins: These proteins are necessary for muscle repair, metabolism, and satiety. Gastric sleeve patients should eat lean proteins such skinless poultry, fish, shellfish, tofu, tempeh, beans, lentils, and low-fat dairy products.

2. Non-Starchy veggies: Non-starchy veggies are low in calories but high in fiber, vitamins, and minerals, making them perfect for gastric sleeve patients. Incorporate a variety of colorful veggies into your meals, such as leafy greens, broccoli, cauliflower, bell peppers, zucchini, spinach, and tomatoes, to boost nutrition and flavor.

3. Whole Grains: Whole grains include complex carbs, fiber, and important minerals that promote energy and digestive health. Choose whole grains like quinoa, brown rice, oats, barley, bulgur, and whole wheat pasta to add texture and nutrition to your dishes.

4. Healthy Fats: While gastric sleeve patients should restrict their fat consumption, eating healthy fats in moderation can benefit heart health, cognitive function, and vitamin absorption. Avocado, almonds, seeds, olive oil, and fatty fish such as salmon and trout are all good sources of healthful fat.

5. Fresh Herbs and Spices: Fresh herbs and spices provide flavor to dishes without adding calories, salt, or fat. To make wonderful, gratifying recipes, try using herbs and spices like basil, cilantro, parsley, rosemary, thyme, garlic, ginger, turmeric, cumin, and paprika.

6. Low-Calorie taste Enhancers: Gastric sleeve patients can add taste to their meals without consuming extra calories by

utilizing low-calorie flavor enhancers such vinegar, citrus juice, mustard, spicy sauce, and salsa. These ingredients may brighten up recipes and make healthy eating more appealing.

7. High-Fiber Foods: Fiber-rich foods are good for your digestive health, blood sugar control, and weight management. Include high-fiber foods in your diet, such as fruits, vegetables, whole grains, legumes, and nuts, to promote fullness and satisfaction while also supporting regular bowel movements.

8. Low-Sugar Condiments and Sauces: Many condiments and sauces contain added sugars, which can lead to excessive calorie intake and weight gain. To limit added sugar in your diet while still eating delectable meals, choose low-sugar or sugar-free versions of condiments such as ketchup, barbecue sauce, salad dressing, and marinades.

9. Low-Calorie Sweeteners: For people with a sweet craving, low-calorie sweeteners can be used sparingly to give sweetness to foods and beverages without adding calories. Stevia, erythritol, and monk fruit extract can help fulfill sweet cravings while without significantly altering blood sugar levels or weight reduction attempts.

10. Hydration Aids: Maintaining hydration is critical for general health and well-being, particularly following gastric sleeve surgery. Keep a supply of hydration aids on hand, like herbal teas, sugar-free drink mixes, flavored water enhancers, and infused water pitchers, to make staying hydrated more fun and simple.

11. Individualized Supplements: Depending on their nutritional demands and any deficiencies discovered by healthcare specialists, gastric sleeve

patients may benefit from taking specific supplements to help them stay healthy. Multivitamins, calcium, vitamin D, iron, vitamin B12, and omega-3 fatty acids are among the most common supplements. To discover whether supplements are suitable and essential for you, speak with your healthcare physician or a qualified nutritionist.

By filling your kitchen with these essential products, you'll be able to cook tasty, healthy meals that support your health and weight reduction objectives following gastric sleeve surgery. Experiment with varied flavors, textures, and cooking methods to keep meals interesting and pleasant, and don't be afraid to be creative in the kitchen!

To summarize, preparing your kitchen with necessary tools and food is a vital step toward success following gastric sleeve surgery. With the correct equipment and a well-stocked pantry, you'll be able to prepare tasty, healthy meals that help you achieve your health and weight reduction objectives. Remember to prioritize lean meats, non-starchy veggies, whole grains, healthy fats, and flavor-enhancing elements in your cooking. Stay hydrated and supplement as required to meet your nutritional needs. With determination, imagination, and a little culinary flare, you may go on a vivid and satisfying culinary adventure to improve your health and well-being.

CHAPTER 2

Breakfasts for Champions

Protein-Packed Breakfast Ideas

1. Spinach and Feta Omelette

Ingredients:

- - 2 eggs
- - 1 cup fresh spinach, chopped
- - 2 tbsp crumbled feta cheese
- - Salt and pepper to taste

Instructions:

1. In a bowl, whisk together the eggs, salt, and pepper.

2. Heat a non-stick skillet over medium heat and coat with cooking spray.

3. Pour the egg mixture into the skillet and cook for 2-3 minutes until the bottom is set.

4. Sprinkle the chopped spinach and feta cheese over one half of the omelette.

5. Fold the other half of the omelette over the filling and cook for an additional 1-2 minutes until the cheese is melted and the omelette is cooked through.

6. Serve hot.

- Preparation Time: 5 minutes

- Cooking Time: 5 minutes

- Yield: 1 serving

- Nutritional Information (per serving):

- Calories: 260

- Protein: 19g

- Carbohydrates: 3g

- Fat: 19g

- Fiber: 1g

2. Greek Yogurt Parfait with Berries

Ingredients:

- - 1/2 cup Greek yogurt
- - 1/4 cup fresh berries (e.g., strawberries, blueberries, raspberries)
- - 2 tbsp granola
- - 1 tsp honey (optional)

- Instructions:
- 1. In a glass or bowl, layer the Greek yogurt, fresh berries, and granola.
- 2. Drizzle honey over the top if desired.
- 3. Serve immediately.
-
- - Preparation Time: 5 minutes
- - Cooking Time: 0 minutes
- - Yield: 1 serving
- - Nutritional Information (per serving):
- - Calories: 200
- - Protein: 15g
- - Carbohydrates: 25g
- - Fat: 6g
- - Fiber: 3g

3. Protein Pancakes with Maple Syrup

- Ingredients:

- - 1/2 cup rolled oats
- - 1/2 cup cottage cheese
- - 2 eggs
- - 1/2 tsp vanilla extract
- - 1/4 tsp cinnamon
- - Cooking spray
- - Sugar-free maple syrup for serving

- Instructions:

- 1. In a blender, combine the rolled oats, cottage cheese, eggs, vanilla extract, and cinnamon. Blend until smooth.
- 2. Heat a non-stick skillet over medium heat and coat with cooking spray.
- 3. Pour small portions of the pancake batter onto the skillet and cook for 2-3 minutes on each side until golden brown.
- 4. Serve the pancakes with sugar-free maple syrup.
-
- - Preparation Time: 10 minutes
- - Cooking Time: 5 minutes
- - Yield: 2 servings (4 small pancakes)
- - Nutritional Information (per serving, without syrup):

- - Calories: 220

- Protein: 17g

- Carbohydrates: 17g

- Fat: 9g

- Fiber: 2g

4. Breakfast Egg Muffins

- **Ingredients:**

  - 6 eggs

  - 1/2 cup diced bell peppers

  - 1/2 cup diced tomatoes

  - 1/4 cup diced onions

  - 1/4 cup shredded cheese

  - Salt and pepper to taste

- **Instructions:**

  - 1. Preheat the oven to 350°F (175°C) and grease a muffin tin with cooking spray.
  - 2. In a bowl, whisk together the eggs, salt, and pepper.
  - 3. Divide the diced vegetables and shredded cheese evenly among the muffin cups.
  - 4. Pour the egg mixture over the vegetables and cheese, filling each muffin cup about 3/4 full.
  - 5. Bake for 20-25 minutes until the egg muffins are set and lightly golden.
  - 6. Allow the egg muffins to cool slightly before removing them from the muffin tin.
  - 7. Serve warm or refrigerate for later use.
  - - Preparation Time: 10 minutes
  - - Cooking Time: 20-25 minutes
  - - Yield: 6 servings (2 egg muffins per serving)
  - - Nutritional Information (per serving):
  - - Calories: 120
  - - Protein: 10g
  - - Carbohydrates: 3g
  - - Fat: 7g
  - - Fiber: 1gQuick and Easy Breakfast Options

5. Avocado Toast with Poached Egg

- Ingredients:

- 1 slice whole grain bread

- 1/2 ripe avocado, mashed

- 1 poached egg

- Salt and pepper to taste

Instructions:

- 1. Toast the slice of whole grain bread until golden brown.
- 2. Spread the mashed avocado evenly over the toasted bread.
- 3. Top with a poached egg and season with salt and pepper to taste.
- 4. Serve immediately.
-
- - Preparation Time: 10 minutes
- - Cooking Time: 5 minutes
- - Yield: 1 serving
- - Nutritional Information (per serving):
- - Calories: 250
- - Protein: 12g
- - Carbohydrates: 17g
- - Fat: 16g
- - Fiber: 7g

6. Cottage Cheese Pancakes

Ingredients:

- 1/2 cup low-fat cottage cheese

- 2 eggs

- 1/4 cup rolled oats

- 1/2 tsp vanilla extract

- Cooking spray

- **Instructions**:
- 1. In a blender, combine the cottage cheese, eggs, rolled oats, and vanilla extract. Blend until smooth.
- 2. Heat a non-stick skillet over medium heat and coat with cooking spray.
- 3. Pour small portions of the pancake batter onto the skillet and cook for 2-3 minutes on each side until golden brown.
- 4. Serve the pancakes with your favorite toppings such as fresh fruit, honey, or sugar-free syrup.

- - Preparation Time: 10 minutes
- - Cooking Time: 5 minutes
- - Yield: 2 servings (4 small pancakes)
- - Nutritional Information (per serving):
- - Calories: 200
- - Protein: 18g
- - Carbohydrates: 12g
- - Fat: 8g
- - Fiber: 2g

7. Overnight Oats with Chia Seeds

- Ingredients:

- - 1/2 cup rolled oats
- - 1/2 cup unsweetened almond milk
- - 1 tbsp chia seeds
- - 1/2 tsp vanilla extract
- - 1/4 cup fresh berries (optional)
- - 1 tsp honey or maple syrup (optional)

Instructions:

- 1. In a mason jar or container, combine the rolled oats, almond milk, chia seeds, and vanilla extract. Stir well to combine.
- 2. Cover the jar and refrigerate overnight or for at least 4 hours to allow the oats and chia seeds to absorb the liquid and soften.
- 3. Before serving, stir the mixture and top with fresh berries and a drizzle of honey or maple syrup if desired.
- - Preparation Time: 5 minutes
- - Cooking Time: 0 minutes (overnight refrigeration)
- - Yield: 1 serving
- - Nutritional Information (per serving):
- - Calories: 250
- - Protein: 8g
- - Carbohydrates: 36g
- - Fat: 9g
- - Fiber: 9g

8. Breakfast Quesadillas

- **Ingredients**:

- 2 small whole grain tortillas

- 2 eggs, scrambled

- 1/4 cup shredded cheese

- 1/4 cup diced bell peppers

- 1/4 cup diced onions

- 1/4 cup salsa

- Cooking spray

Instructions:

1. Heat a non-stick skillet over medium heat and coat with cooking spray.

2. Place one tortilla in the skillet and top with scrambled eggs, shredded cheese, diced bell peppers, and onions.

3. Place the second tortilla on top and press down gently to seal.

4. Cook for 2-3 minutes on each side until the tortillas are golden brown and the cheese is melted.

5. Cut the quesadilla into wedges and serve with salsa for dipping.

- - Preparation Time: 10 minutes
- - Cooking Time: 5 minutes
- - Yield: 1 serving
- - Nutritional Information (per serving):
- - Calories: 400
- - Protein: 24g
- - Carbohydrates: 30g
- - Fat: 20g
- - Fiber: 6g

Make-Ahead Breakfasts for Busy Mornings

9. Overnight Chia Seed Pudding

- **Ingredients:**

- - 2 tbsp chia seeds
- - 1/2 cup unsweetened almond milk
- - 1/4 tsp vanilla extract
- - 1/4 cup fresh fruit (e.g., berries, sliced banana)
- - 1 tbsp chopped nuts or seeds (optional)
- - 1 tsp honey or maple syrup (optional)

- Instructions:

1. In a mason jar or container, combine the chia seeds, almond milk, and vanilla extract. Stir well to combine.

2. Cover the jar and refrigerate overnight or for at least 4 hours to allow the chia seeds to absorb the liquid and thicken.

3. Before serving, stir the mixture and top with fresh fruit, chopped nuts or seeds, and a drizzle of honey or maple syrup if desired.

- Preparation Time: 5 minutes
- Cooking Time: 0 minutes (overnight refrigeration)
- Yield: 1 serving
- Nutritional Information (per serving):
- Calories: 150
- Protein: 5g
- Carbohydrates: 15g
- Fat: 9g
- Fiber: 10g

10. Breakfast Burrito Bowls

- Ingredients:

- - 1/2 cup cooked quinoa or brown rice
- - 1/4 cup black beans, drained and rinsed
- - 1/4 cup diced bell peppers
- - 1/4 cup diced tomatoes
- - 1/4 cup diced avocado
- -1. Breakfast Burrito Bowls
- - 1/4 cup cooked lean ground turkey or chicken
- - 1/4 cup shredded cheese
- - 1 egg, cooked to preference (optional)
- - Salsa, for serving
- - Fresh cilantro, for garnish (optional)

Instructions:

1. In a bowl, layer the cooked quinoa or brown rice, black beans, diced bell peppers, diced tomatoes, diced avocado, and cooked lean ground turkey or chicken.

2. Top with shredded cheese and a cooked egg if desired.

3. Serve with salsa on the side and garnish with fresh cilantro if desired.

4. Mix well before eating.

- - Preparation Time: 15 minutes
- - Cooking Time: 10 minutes
- - Yield: 1 serving
- - Nutritional Information (per serving):
- - Calories: 400
- - Protein: 30g
- - Carbohydrates: 30g
- - Fat: 18g
- - Fiber: 8g

2. Veggie Egg Casserole

- Ingredients:

- 6 eggs

- 1/2 cup diced bell peppers

- 1/2 cup diced onions

- 1/2 cup diced tomatoes

- 1 cup chopped spinach

- 1/4 cup shredded cheese

- Salt and pepper to taste

- Cooking spray

Instructions:

1. Preheat the oven to 350°F (175°C) and grease a baking dish with cooking spray.

2. In a bowl, whisk together the eggs, salt, and pepper.

3. Stir in the diced bell peppers, onions, tomatoes, chopped spinach, and shredded cheese.

4. Pour the egg mixture into the prepared baking dish.

5. Bake for 25-30 minutes until the egg casserole is set and lightly golden on top.

6. Allow to cool slightly before slicing and serving.

- - Preparation Time: 15 minutes
- - Cooking Time: 25-30 minutes
- - Yield: 4 servings
- - Nutritional Information (per serving):
- - Calories: 150
- - Protein: 12g
- - Carbohydrates: 6g
- - Fat: 8g
- - Fiber: 2g

3. Banana Bread Breakfast Bars

- Ingredients:

- - 2 ripe bananas, mashed
- - 1/4 cup almond butter
- - 1/4 cup honey or maple syrup
- - 1 tsp vanilla extract
- - 1 1/2 cups rolled oats
- - 1/4 cup chopped nuts or seeds (e.g., walnuts, almonds, pumpkin seeds)
- - 1/4 cup dried fruit (e.g., raisins, cranberries, chopped dates)
- - 1/2 tsp cinnamon
- - Pinch of salt

Instructions:

1. Preheat the oven to 350°F (175°C) and grease a baking dish with cooking spray.

2. In a large bowl, combine the mashed bananas, almond butter, honey or maple syrup, and vanilla extract. Mix well.

3. Stir in the rolled oats, chopped nuts or seeds, dried fruit, cinnamon, and salt until well combined.

4. Press the mixture evenly into the prepared baking dish.

5. Bake for 25-30 minutes until golden brown and set.

6. Allow to cool completely before cutting into bars.

- - Preparation Time: 10 minutes
- - Cooking Time: 25-30 minutes
- - Yield: 12 bars
- - Nutritional Information (per bar):
- - Calories: 150
- - Protein: 3g
- - Carbohydrates: 20g
- - Fat: 7g
- - Fiber: 3g

CHAPTER 3

Satisfying Soups and Salads

Nourishing Soup Recipes

1. Butternut Squash Soup

- Ingredients:

- - 1 medium butternut squash, peeled, seeded, and cubed
- - 1 onion, diced
- - 2 cloves garlic, minced
- - 4 cups vegetable or chicken broth
- - 1 tsp dried thyme
- - Salt and pepper to taste
- - Optional toppings: Greek yogurt, pumpkin seeds, chopped fresh herbs

Instructions:

1. In a large pot, heat olive oil over medium heat. Add the diced onion and garlic, and sauté until softened, about 5 minutes.

2. Add the cubed butternut squash, vegetable or chicken broth, and dried thyme to the pot. Bring to a boil, then reduce heat and simmer for 20-25 minutes, until the squash is tender.

3. Use an immersion blender to puree the soup until smooth. Alternatively, transfer the soup in batches to a blender and blend until smooth, then return to the pot.

4. Season with salt and pepper to taste. Serve hot, garnished with optional toppings if desired.

- - Preparation Time: 15 minutes
- - Cooking Time: 25 minutes
- - Yield: 4 servings
- - Nutritional Information (per serving):
- - Calories: 120
- - Protein: 2g
- - Carbohydrates: 28g
- - Fat: 1g
- - Fiber: 5g

2. Chicken and Vegetable Soup

- Ingredients:

- 1 tbsp olive oil

- 1 onion, diced

- 2 carrots, diced

- 2 celery stalks, diced

- 2 cloves garlic, minced

- 4 cups chicken broth

- 2 cups cooked shredded chicken breast

- 1 cup diced tomatoes

- 1 tsp dried thyme

- Salt and pepper to taste

- Optional garnish: chopped fresh parsley

Instructions:

1. In a large pot, heat olive oil over medium heat. Add the diced onion, carrots, and celery, and sauté until softened, about 5 minutes.

2. Add the minced garlic to the pot and cook for an additional minute until fragrant.

3. Pour in the chicken broth, shredded chicken breast, diced tomatoes, and dried thyme. Bring to a boil, then reduce heat and simmer for 20-25 minutes.

4. Season with salt and pepper to taste. Serve hot, garnished with chopped fresh parsley if desired.

- - Preparation Time: 15 minutes
- - Cooking Time: 25 minutes
- - Yield: 4 servings
- - Nutritional Information (per serving):
- - Calories: 180
- - Protein: 20g
- - Carbohydrates: 10g
- - Fat: 7g
- - Fiber: 2g

3. Lentil Soup

Ingredients:

- 1 tbsp olive oil

- 1 onion, diced

- 2 carrots, diced

- 2 celery stalks, diced

- 2 cloves garlic, minced

- 1 cup dried lentils, rinsed and drained

- 4 cups vegetable or chicken broth

- 1 tsp ground cumin

- 1/2 tsp paprika

- Salt and pepper to taste

- Optional garnish: chopped fresh cilantro or parsley

Instructions:

1. In a large pot, heat olive oil over medium heat. Add the diced onion, carrots, and celery, and sauté until softened, about 5 minutes.

2. Add the minced garlic to the pot and cook for an additional minute until fragrant

3. Add the dried lentils, vegetable or chicken broth, ground cumin, and paprika to the pot. Bring to a boil, then reduce heat and simmer for 20-25 minutes, until the lentils are tender.

4. Season with salt and pepper to taste. Serve hot, garnished with chopped fresh cilantro or parsley if desired.

- - Preparation Time: 15 minutes
- - Cooking Time: 25 minutes
- - Yield: 4 servings
- - Nutritional Information (per serving):
- - Calories: 220
- - Protein: 12g
- - Carbohydrates: 35g
- - Fat: 4g
- - Fiber: 15g

4. Creamy Tomato Basil Soup

- **Ingredients:**
- - 1 tbsp olive oil
- - 1 onion, diced
- - 2 cloves garlic, minced
- - 2 cans (14 oz each) diced tomatoes
- - 2 cups vegetable or chicken broth
- - 1/2 cup fresh basil leaves, chopped

- - 1/2 cup heavy cream or coconut milk
- - Salt and pepper to taste
- - Optional garnish: fresh basil leaves, grated Parmesan cheese

Instructions:

1. In a large pot, heat olive oil over medium heat. Add the diced onion and garlic, and sauté until softened, about 5 minutes.

2. Add the diced tomatoes (with their juices) and vegetable or chicken broth to the pot. Bring to a boil, then reduce heat and simmer for 15-20 minutes.

3. Stir in the chopped fresh basil leaves and heavy cream or coconut milk. Simmer for an additional 5 minutes.

4. Use an immersion blender to puree the soup until smooth. Alternatively, transfer the soup in batches to a blender and blend until smooth, then return to the pot.

5. Season with salt and pepper to taste. Serve hot, garnished with fresh basil leaves and grated Parmesan cheese if desired.

- - Preparation Time: 10 minutes
- - Cooking Time: 25 minutes
- - Yield: 4 servings
- - Nutritional Information (per serving):
- - Calories: 250
- - Protein: 6g
- - Carbohydrates: 20g
- - Fat: 16g
- - Fiber: 5g

Refreshing Salad Creations

5. Grilled Chicken Caesar Salad

Ingredients:

- - 2 boneless, skinless chicken breasts
- - 1 tbsp olive oil
- - Salt and pepper to taste

- - 4 cups romaine lettuce, chopped
- - 1/4 cup grated Parmesan cheese
- - 1/2 cup Caesar salad dressing (store-bought or homemade)
- - Croutons for serving (optional)

Instructions:

1. Preheat the grill or grill pan over medium-high heat.

2. Season chicken breasts with olive oil, salt, and pepper.

3. Grill chicken for 6-7 minutes per side, or until cooked through and no longer pink in the center.

4. Let the chicken rest for a few minutes, then slice it thinly.

5. In a large bowl, toss the chopped romaine lettuce with Caesar dressing until well coated.

6. Divide the dressed lettuce among serving plates and top with sliced grilled chicken.

7. Sprinkle grated Parmesan cheese over the top and serve immediately, garnished with croutons if desired.

- - Preparation Time: 10 minutes
- - Cooking Time: 15 minutes
- - Yield: 2 servings
- - Nutritional Information (per serving):
- - Calories: 400
- - Protein: 35g
- - Carbohydrates: 10g
- - Fat: 25g
- - Fiber: 3g

6. Mediterranean Quinoa Salad

Ingredients:

- - 1 cup cooked quinoa
- - 1 cup cherry tomatoes, halved
- - 1 cucumber, diced
- - 1/2 cup Kalamata olives, pitted and halved
- - 1/4 cup red onion, thinly sliced

- - 1/4 cup crumbled feta cheese
- - 2 tbsp chopped fresh parsley
- - 2 tbsp extra virgin olive oil
- - 1 tbsp lemon juice
- - Salt and pepper to taste

Instructions:

1. In a large bowl, combine the cooked quinoa, cherry tomatoes, cucumber, Kalamata olives, red onion, feta cheese, and parsley.

2. Drizzle with extra virgin olive oil and lemon juice.

3. Season with salt and pepper to taste.

4. Toss until all ingredients are well combined

5. Serve immediately, or refrigerate until ready to serve.

- - Preparation Time: 15 minutes
- - Cooking Time: 15 minutes (for cooking quinoa)
- - Yield: 4 servings

- - Nutritional Information (per serving):
- - Calories: 250
- - Protein: 6g
- - Carbohydrates: 25g
- - Fat: 15g
- - Fiber: 4g

7. Thai Beef Salad

Ingredients:

- 8 oz flank steak

- 2 tbsp soy sauce

- 1 tbsp fish sauce

- 1 tbsp lime juice

- 1 tsp honey

- 1 clove garlic, minced

- 1/2 tsp grated ginger

- 4 cups mixed salad greens

- 1/2 cucumber, thinly sliced

- 1/2 cup cherry tomatoes, halved

- 1/4 cup thinly sliced red onion

- 1/4 cup chopped fresh cilantro

- 1/4 cup chopped fresh mint

- Optional garnish: chopped peanuts, lime wedges

Instructions:

1. Preheat the grill or grill pan over medium-high heat.

2. In a small bowl, whisk together soy sauce, fish sauce, lime juice, honey, garlic, and ginger to make the marinade.

3. Place flank steak in a shallow dish and pour marinade over it. Let it marinate for at least 30 minutes.

4. Grill steak for 3-4 minutes per side, or until desired doneness. Let it rest for a few minutes, then slice thinly against the grain.

5. In a large bowl, toss mixed salad greens, cucumber, cherry tomatoes, red onion, cilantro, and mint.

6. Divide salad among serving plates and top with sliced grilled steak.

7. Garnish with chopped peanuts and lime wedges if desired. Serve immediately.

- - Preparation Time: 40 minutes (including marination time)
- - Cooking Time: 8 minutes
- - Yield: 2 servings
- - Nutritional Information (per serving):
- - Calories: 350
- - Protein: 30g
- - Carbohydrates: 15g
- - Fat: 18g
- - Fiber: 4g

8. Caprese Salad

- Ingredients:

- 2 large ripe tomatoes, sliced

- 1 ball fresh mozzarella cheese, sliced

- 1/4 cup fresh basil leaves

- 2 tbsp balsamic glaze

- 1 tbsp extra virgin olive oil

- Salt and pepper to taste

Instructions:

1. Arrange sliced tomatoes and fresh mozzarella cheese on a serving platter, alternating them.

2. Tuck fresh basil leaves in between the tomato and mozzarella slices.3. Drizzle balsamic glaze and extra virgin olive oil over the top.

4. Season with salt and pepper to taste.

5. Serve immediately, or refrigerate until ready to serve.

- - Preparation Time: 10 minutes
- - Cooking Time: 0 minutes
- - Yield: 2 servings
- - Nutritional Information (per serving):
- - Calories: 250
- - Protein: 15g
- - Carbohydrates: 10g
- - Fat: 18g
- - Fiber: 2g

Tips for Creating Balanced and Filling Soups and Salads

Creating balanced and filling soups and salads involves incorporating a variety of nutritious ingredients such as lean proteins, whole grains, healthy fats, and plenty of vegetables. Here are some tips to help you create satisfying meals:

- **Start with a base**: Choose nutrient-rich bases for your soups and salads, such as quinoa, brown rice, lentils, or leafy greens.

- **Add protein:** Include lean proteins such as chicken breast, turkey, tofu, beans, or lentils to help keep you feeling full and satisfied.

- **Load up on vegetables:** Pack your soups and salads with a variety of colorful vegetables for added fiber, vitamins, and minerals.

- **Don't forget healthy fats**: Incorporate sources of healthy fats such as avocado, nuts, seeds, or olive oil to add flavor and promote satiety.

- **Use flavorful seasonings:** Enhance the taste of your soups and salads with herbs, spices, citrus juice, and vinegar instead of relying on excess salt or sugar.

- **Watch portion sizes**: Be mindful of portion sizes to avoid overeating, especially when it comes to higher-calorie ingredients like cheese, nuts, and dressings.

- Experiment with textures: Add crunch to your salads with nuts, seeds, or crispy vegetables, and vary the texture of your soups with ingredients like beans or whole grains.

Flavorful Chicken Recipes

1. Lemon Herb Roast Chicken

- Ingredients:

- 1 whole chicken (about 4 lbs)

- 2 tbsp olive oil

- 2 cloves garlic, minced

- 1 lemon, sliced

- 2 tbsp fresh herbs (such as rosemary, thyme, or parsley), chopped

- Salt and pepper to taste

Instructions:

1. Preheat the oven to 375°F (190°C).

2. Rinse the chicken and pat it dry with paper towels. Place it in a roasting pan.

3. In a small bowl, mix together olive oil, minced garlic, chopped herbs, salt, and pepper.

4. Rub the olive oil mixture all over the chicken, including under the skin.

5. Stuff the cavity of the chicken with lemon slices.

6. Roast the chicken in the preheated oven for 1 to 1 1/2 hours, or until the internal temperature reaches 165°F (75°C) and the juices run clear.

7. Let the chicken rest for 10 minutes before carving. Serve hot.

- - Preparation Time: 15 minutes
- - Cooking Time: 1 to 1 1/2 hours
- - Yield: 4 servings
- - Nutritional Information (per serving):
- - Calories: 300
- - Protein: 30g
- - Carbohydrates: 2g
- - Fat: 18g
- - Fiber: 1g

2. Chicken Stir-Fry with Veggies

Ingredients:

- 2 boneless, skinless chicken breasts, sliced

- 2 tbsp soy sauce

- 1 tbsp hoisin sauce

- 1 tbsp oyster sauce

- 1 tbsp sesame oil

- 2 cloves garlic, minced

- 1 inch ginger, grated

- 2 cups mixed vegetables (such as bell peppers, broccoli, carrots, snap peas)

- Cooked rice or quinoa, for serving

- Optional garnish: sliced green onions, sesame seeds

Instructions:

1. In a bowl, combine sliced chicken breast with soy sauce, hoisin sauce, and oyster sauce. Let it marinate for 15-20 minutes.

2. Heat sesame oil in a large skillet or wok over medium-high heat.

3. Add minced garlic and grated ginger to the skillet and sauté for 1 minute until fragrant.

4. Add marinated chicken to the skillet and stir-fry for 5-6 minutes until cooked through.

5. Add mixed vegetables to the skillet and continue to stir-fry for another 3-4 minutes until vegetables are tender-crisp.

6. Serve chicken stir-fry hot over cooked rice or quinoa. Garnish with sliced green onions and sesame seeds if desired.

- Preparation Time: 20 minutes
- Cooking Time: 15 minutes
- Yield: 4 servings
- Nutritional Information (per serving):
- Calories: 250
- Protein: 25g
- Carbohydrates: 15g
- Fat: 10g
- Fiber: 4g

3. Chicken and Broccoli Casserole

Ingredients:

- - 2 boneless, skinless chicken breasts, cooked and shredded
- - 2 cups cooked quinoa or brown rice
- - 2 cups broccoli florets, steamed
- - 1 cup shredded cheddar cheese
- - 1/2 cup plain Greek yogurt
- - 1/4 cup milk
- - 2 cloves garlic, minced
- - 1 tsp dried thyme
- - Salt and pepper to taste
- - Cooking spray

Instructions:

1. Preheat the oven to 375°F (190°C). Grease a casserole dish with cooking spray.

2. In a large bowl, combine shredded chicken, cooked quinoa or brown rice, steamed broccoli florets, and shredded cheddar cheese. Mix well.

3. In a separate bowl, whisk together Greek yogurt, milk, minced garlic, dried thyme, salt, and pepper.

4. Pour the yogurt mixture over the chicken and broccoli mixture, and stir until everything is evenly coated.

5. Transfer the mixture to the prepared casserole dish and spread it out evenly.

6. Bake in the preheated oven for 20-25 minutes, until the cheese is melted and bubbly.

7. Serve hot.

- - Preparation Time: 20 minutes
- - Cooking Time: 25 minutes
- - Yield: 4 servings
- - Nutritional Information (per serving):
- - Calories: 350
- - Protein: 30g
- - Carbohydrates: 25g
- - Fat: 15g
- - Fiber: 4g

4. Grilled Chicken Skewers with Peanut Sauce

Ingredients:

- 2 boneless, skinless chicken breasts, cut into cubes

- Wooden skewers, soaked in water for 30 minutes

- 1/4 cup peanut butter

- 2 tbsp soy sauce

- 1 tbsp honey

- 1 tbsp rice vinegar

- 1 clove garlic, minced

- 1/2 tsp grated ginger

- Pinch of red pepper flakes (optional)

- Chopped peanuts and sliced green onions for garnish (optional)

Instructions:

1. Preheat the grill or grill pan over medium-high heat.

2. Thread chicken cubes onto soaked wooden skewers.

3. In a small saucepan, combine peanut butter, soy sauce, honey, rice vinegar, minced garlic, grated ginger, and red pepper flakes (if using). Heat over low heat, stirring until smooth and well combined

4. Grill chicken skewers for 4-5 minutes per side, or until cooked through and lightly charred.

5. Serve grilled chicken skewers hot with peanut sauce drizzled on top. Garnish with chopped peanuts and sliced green onions if desired.

- - Preparation Time: 15 minutes
- - Cooking Time: 10 minutes
- - Yield: 4 servings
- - Nutritional Information (per serving):
- - Calories: 300
- - Protein: 25g
- - Carbohydrates: 10g
- - Fat: 15g
- - Fiber: 2g

5. Baked Salmon with Dill Sauce

- Ingredients:

  - 4 salmon fillets

  - 2 tbsp olive oil

  - Salt and pepper to taste

  - 1/4 cup plain Greek yogurt

  - 1 tbsp lemon juice

  - 1 tbsp chopped fresh dill

  - 1 clove garlic, minced

  - Lemon wedges for serving

Instructions:

1. Preheat the oven to 375°F (190°C). Line a baking sheet with parchment paper.

2. Place salmon filets on the prepared baking sheet. Drizzle with olive oil and season with salt and pepper.

3. Bake in the preheated oven for 12-15 minutes, or until salmon is cooked through and flakes easily with a fork.

4. While the salmon is baking, prepare the dill sauce. In a small bowl, whisk together Greek yogurt, lemon juice, chopped fresh dill, and minced garlic until well combined.

5. Serve baked salmon hot, with dill sauce drizzled on top and lemon wedges on the side.

- - Preparation Time: 10 minutes
- - Cooking Time: 12-15 minutes
- - Yield: 4 servings
- - Nutritional Information (per serving):
- - Calories: 250
- - Protein: 25g
- - Carbohydrates: 2g
- - Fat: 15g
- - Fiber: 0g

6. Shrimp and Veggie Stir-Fry

Ingredients:

- 1 lb large shrimp, peeled and deveined

- 2 tbsp soy sauce

- 1 tbsp oyster sauce

- 1 tbsp hoisin sauce

- 1 tbsp sesame oil

- 2 cloves garlic, minced

- 1 inch ginger, grated

- 2 cups mixed vegetables (such as bell peppers, snap peas, carrots, broccoli)

- Cooked rice or noodles, for serving

- Optional garnish: sliced green onions, sesame seeds

Instructions:

1. In a bowl, combine shrimp with soy sauce, oyster sauce, and hoisin sauce. Let it marinate for 15-20 minutes.

2. Heat sesame oil in a large skillet or wok over medium-high heat.

3. Add minced garlic and grated ginger to the skillet and sauté for 1 minute until fragrant.

4. Add marinated shrimp to the skillet and stir-fry for 2-3 minutes until pink and cooked through. Remove shrimp from the skillet and set aside.

5. In the same skillet, add mixed vegetables and stir-fry for 3-4 minutes until tender-crisp.

6. Return cooked shrimp to the skillet and toss everything together until well combined.

7. Serve shrimp and veggie stir-fry hot over cooked rice or noodles. Garnish with sliced green onions and sesame seeds if desired.

- Preparation Time: 20 minutes
- Cooking Time: 10 minutes
- Yield: 4 servings
- Nutritional Information (per serving):
- Calories: 200
- Protein: 20g
- Carbohydrates: 15g
- Fat: 8g
- Fiber: 3g

7. Garlic Butter Grilled Shrimp

Ingredients:

- - 1 lb large shrimp, peeled and deveined
- - 2 tbsp unsalted butter, melted
- - 2 cloves garlic, minced
- - 1 tbsp chopped fresh parsley
- - Salt and pepper to taste
- - Lemon wedges for serving

Instructions:

1. Preheat grill or grill pan over medium-high heat.

2. In a bowl, combine melted butter, minced garlic, chopped fresh parsley, salt, and pepper.

3. Thread shrimp onto skewers.

4. Grill shrimp skewers for 2-3 minutes per side, or until pink and cooked through.

5. Remove shrimp skewers from the grill and brush with garlic butter mixture.

6. Serve grilled shrimp hot, with lemon wedges on the side.

- - Preparation Time: 10 minutes
- - Cooking Time: 6 minutes
- - Yield: 4 servings
- - Nutritional Information (per serving):
- - Calories: 150
- - Protein: 25g
- - Carbohydrates: 1g
- - Fat: 6g
- - Fiber: 0g

8. Lemon Herb Baked Cod

- Ingredients:

- 4 cod fillets

- 2 tbsp olive oil

- 2 tbsp lemon juice

- 1 tbsp chopped fresh dill

- 1 tbsp chopped fresh parsley

- 2 cloves garlic, minced

- Salt and pepper to taste

- Lemon wedges for serving

Instructions:

1. Preheat the oven to 400°F (200°C). Line a baking sheet with parchment paper.

2. Place cod fillets on the prepared baking sheet. Drizzle with olive oil and lemon juice.

3. Sprinkle chopped fresh dill, chopped fresh parsley, minced garlic, salt, and pepper over the cod fillets.

4. Bake in the preheated oven for 12-15 minutes, or until the cod is opaque and flakes easily with a fork.

5. Serve baked cod hot, with lemon wedges on the side.

- - Preparation Time: 10 minutes
- - Cooking Time: 12-15 minutes
- - Yield: 4 servings
- - Nutritional Information (per serving):
- - Calories: 200
- - Protein: 25g
- - Carbohydrates: 1g
- - Fat: 10g
- - Fiber: 0g

Lean Meat Innovations

9. Turkey and Veggie Meatballs

- **Ingredients:**

  - 1 lb ground turkey

  - 1/2 cup grated zucchini

  - 1/2 cup grated carrot

  - 1/4 cup chopped fresh parsley

  - 1/4 cup breadcrumbs

  - 1 egg

  - 2 cloves garlic, minced

  - 1 tsp Italian seasoning

  - Salt and pepper to taste

  - Cooking spray

Instructions:

1. Preheat the oven to 375°F (190°C). Line a baking sheet with parchment paper and lightly grease with cooking spray.

2. In a largebowl, combine ground turkey, grated zucchini, grated carrot, chopped fresh parsley, breadcrumbs, egg,

minced garlic, Italian seasoning, salt, and pepper. Mix until well combined.

3. Shape the mixture into meatballs, using about 1-2 tablespoons of mixture for each meatball, and place them on the prepared baking sheet.

4. Bake in the preheated oven for 20-25 minutes, or until meatballs are cooked through and lightly browned.

5. Serve turkey and veggie meatballs hot with your favorite sauce or over pasta, rice, or quinoa.

- - Preparation Time: 15 minutes
- - Cooking Time: 20-25 minutes
- - Yield: 4 servings
- - Nutritional Information (per serving):
- - Calories: 250
- - Protein: 25g
- - Carbohydrates: 10g
- - Fat: 12g
- - Fiber: 2g

10. Pork Tenderloin with Apple Chutney

Ingredients:

- 1 lb pork tenderloin

- 1 tbsp olive oil

- Salt and pepper to taste

- For the apple chutney:

  - 2 apples, peeled, cored, and chopped

- 1/4 cup chopped red onion

- 2 tbsp apple cider vinegar

- 2 tbsp honey

- 1/4 tsp ground cinnamon

- Pinch of ground cloves

- Pinch of salt

Instructions:

1. Preheat the oven to 400°F (200°C).

2. Season pork tenderloin with salt and pepper.

3. Heat olive oil in an oven-safe skillet over medium-high heat. Sear the pork tenderloin on all

sides until browned, about 2-3 minutes per side.

4. Transfer the skillet to the preheated oven and roast the pork tenderloin for 15-20 minutes, or until it reaches an internal temperature of 145°F (63°C).

5. While the pork is roasting, prepare the apple chutney. In a saucepan, combine chopped apples, chopped red onion, apple cider vinegar, honey, ground cinnamon, ground cloves, and salt. Cook over medium heat for 10-15 minutes, or until apples are soft and the mixture has thickened.

6. Remove the pork tenderloin from the oven and let it rest for 5 minutes before slicing.

7. Serve sliced pork tenderloin hot with apple chutney spooned over the top.

- - Preparation Time: 15 minutes
- - Cooking Time: 25-30 minutes
- - Yield: 4 servings

- - Nutritional Information (per serving):
- - Calories: 300
- - Protein: 25g
- - Carbohydrates: 20g
- - Fat: 12g
- - Fiber: 2g

11. Beef and Veggie Stir-Fry

Ingredients:

- 1 lb beef sirloin, thinly sliced

- 2 tbsp soy sauce

- 1 tbsp oyster sauce

- 1 tbsp hoisin sauce

- 1 tbsp sesame oil

- 2 cloves garlic, minced

- 1 inch ginger, grated

- 2 cups mixed vegetables (such as bell peppers, broccoli, snap peas, carrots)

- Cooked rice or noodles, for serving

- Optional garnish: sliced green onions, sesame seeds

Instructions:

1. In a bowl, combine sliced beef sirloin with soy sauce, oyster sauce, and hoisin sauce. Let it marinate for 15-20 minutes.

2. Heat sesame oil in a large skillet or wok over medium-high heat.

3. Add minced garlic and grated ginger to the skillet and sauté for 1 minute until fragrant.

4. Add marinated beef sirloin to the skillet and stir-fry for 2-3 minutes until browned.

5. Add mixed vegetables to the skillet and continue to stir-fry for another 3-4 minutes until vegetables are tender-crisp.

6. Serve beef and veggie stir-fry hot over cooked rice or noodles. Garnish with sliced green onions and sesame seeds if desired.

-
-     - Preparation Time: 20 minutes
-     - Cooking Time: 10 minutes
-     - Yield: 4 servings

- - Nutritional Information (per serving):
- - Calories: 300
- - Protein: 30g
- - Carbohydrates: 15g
- - Fat: 12g
- - Fiber: 3g

12. Turkey Chili

- Ingredients:

- 1 lb ground turkey

- 1 onion, chopped

- 2 cloves garlic, minced

- 1 bell pepper, chopped

- 1 jalapeño pepper, seeded and minced (optional)

- 1 can (15 oz) kidney beans, drained and rinsed

- 1 can (15 oz) black beans, drained and rinsed

- 1 can (14 oz) diced tomatoes

- 1 cup chicken broth

- 2 tbsp tomato paste

- 1 tbsp chili powder

- 1 tsp ground cumin

- Salt and pepper to taste

- Optional toppings: shredded cheese, chopped green onions, Greek yogurt or sour cream, diced avocado

Instructions:

1. Heat olive oil in a large pot or Dutch oven over medium heat. Add chopped onion, minced garlic, chopped bell pepper, and minced jalapeño pepper (if using). Cook until vegetables are softened, about 5-7 minutes.

2. Add ground turkey to the pot and cook until browned, breaking it up with a spoon.

3. Stir in kidney beans, black beans, diced tomatoes, chicken broth, tomato paste, chili powder, and ground cumin. Season with salt and pepper to taste.

4. Bring the chili to a simmer and let it cook for 20-25 minutes, stirring occasionally, until flavors are well combined and chili has thickened.

5. Serve turkey chili hot, topped with your favorite toppings such as shredded cheese, chopped green onions, Greek yogurt or sour cream, and diced avocado.

- - Preparation Time: 15 minutes
- - Cooking Time: 30 minutes
- - Yield: 6 servings
- - Nutritional Information (per serving):
- - Calories: 300
- - Protein: 25g
- - Carbohydrates: 25g
- - Fat: 10g
- - Fiber: 8g

CHAPTER 4

Veggie-Centric Creations: Vibrant Vegetable Stir-Fries

1. Teriyaki Tofu Stir-Fry

- Ingredients:

- 1 block firm tofu, pressed and cubed

- 2 cups mixed vegetables (such as bell peppers, broccoli, snap peas, carrots)

- 1/4 cup teriyaki sauce

- 2 tbsp soy sauce

- 1 tbsp sesame oil

- 2 cloves garlic, minced

- Cooked rice or noodles, for serving

- Optional garnish: sliced green onions, sesame seeds

Instructions:

1. In a large skillet or wok, heat sesame oil over medium-high heat.

2. Add cubed tofu to the skillet and cook until golden brown on all sides, about 5-7 minutes. Remove tofu from the skillet and set aside.

3. In the same skillet, add minced garlic and mixed vegetables. Stir-fry for 3-4 minutes until vegetables are tender-crisp.

4. Return cooked tofu to the skillet. Add teriyaki sauce and soy sauce. Stir well to coat everything evenly.

5. Serve teriyaki tofu stir-fry hot over cooked rice or noodles. Garnish with sliced green onions and sesame seeds if desired.

- - Preparation Time: 15 minutes
- - Cooking Time: 15 minutes
- - Yield: 4 servings
- - Nutritional Information (per serving):
- - Calories: 250
- - Protein: 15g
- - Carbohydrates: 20g
- - Fat: 10g
- - Fiber: 4g

2. Stir-Fried Vegetables with Cashews

Ingredients:

- 2 cups mixed vegetables (such as bell peppers, broccoli, snap peas, carrots)

- 1/4 cup cashews

- 2 tbsp soy sauce

- 1 tbsp hoisin sauce

- 1 tbsp sesame oil

- 2 cloves garlic, minced

- Cooked rice or noodles, for serving

- Optional garnish: sliced green onions, sesame seeds

Instructions:

1. In a large skillet or wok, heat sesame oil over medium-high heat.

2. Add minced garlic and mixed vegetables to the skillet. Stir-fry for 3-4 minutes until vegetables are tender-crisp.

3. Add cashews to the skillet and continue to stir-fry for another 1-2 minutes until cashews are lightly toasted.

4. Stir in soy sauce and hoisin sauce, and toss everything together until well coated.

5. Serve stir-fried vegetables with cashews hot over cooked rice or noodles. Garnish with sliced green onions and sesame seeds if desired.

- - Preparation Time: 10 minutes
- - Cooking Time: 10 minutes
- - Yield: 4 servings
- - Nutritional Information (per serving):
- - Calories: 200
- - Protein: 8g
- - Carbohydrates: 15g
- - Fat: 12g
- - Fiber: 4g

3. Spicy Thai Basil Eggplant Stir-Fry

- Ingredients:

- 1 large eggplant, diced

- 2 tbsp soy sauce

- 1 tbsp oyster sauce

- 1 tbsp hoisin sauce

- 1 tbsp sesame oil

- 2 cloves garlic, minced

- 1 red chili, thinly sliced (adjust to taste)

- 1 cup fresh basil leaves

- Cooked rice, for serving

- Optional garnish: sliced green onions, chopped peanuts

Instructions:

1. In a large skillet or wok, heat sesame oil over medium-high heat.

2. Add minced garlic and sliced red chili to the skillet. Sauté for 1 minute until fragrant.

3. Add diced eggplant to the skillet and stir-fry for 5-6 minutes until tender.

4. In a small bowl, mix together soy sauce, oyster sauce, and hoisin sauce. Pour the sauce over the eggplant and stir well to combine.

5. Add fresh basil leaves to the skillet and toss everything together until the basil wilts.

6. Serve spicy Thai basil eggplant stir-fry hot over cooked rice. Garnish with sliced green onions and chopped peanuts if desired.

- Preparation Time: 15 minutes
- Cooking Time: 10 minutes
- Yield: 4 servings
- Nutritional Information (per serving):
- Calories: 180
- Protein: 5g
- Carbohydrates: 20g
- Fat: 10g
- Fiber: 8g

4. Broccoli and Mushroom Stir-Fry

Ingredients:

- 2 cups broccoli florets

- 1 cup sliced mushrooms

- 2 tbsp soy sauce

- 1 tbsp oyster sauce

- 1 tbsp sesame oil

- 2 cloves garlic, minced

- Cooked rice or noodles, for serving

- Optional garnish: sliced green onions, sesame seeds

Instructions:

1. In a large skillet or wok, heat sesame oil over medium-high heat.

2. Add minced garlic to the skillet and sauté for 1 minute until fragrant.

3. Add broccoli florets and sliced mushrooms to the skillet. Stir-fry for 4-5 minutes until vegetables are tender-crisp.

4. In a small bowl, mix together soy sauce and oyster sauce. Pour the sauce over the vegetables and stir well to combine.

5. Serve broccoli and mushroom stir-fry hot over cooked rice or noodles. Garnish with sliced green onions and sesame seeds if desired.

- - Preparation Time: 10 minutes
- - Cooking Time: 10 minutes
- - Yield: 4 servings
- - Nutritional Information (per serving):
- - Calories: 150
- - Protein: 6g
- - Carbohydrates: 15g
- - Fat: 8g
- - Fiber: 5g

Roasted Veggie Marvels

5. Balsamic Roasted Brussels Sprouts

Ingredients:

- 1 lb Brussels sprouts, trimmed and halved

- 2 tbsp olive oil

- 2 tbsp balsamic vinegar

- 1 tbsp honey

- 2 cloves garlic, minced

- Salt and pepper to taste

- Optional garnish: grated Parmesan cheese, chopped parsley

Instructions:

1. Preheat the oven to 400°F (200°C). Line a baking sheet with parchment paper.

2. In a large bowl, toss Brussels sprouts with olive oil, balsamic vinegar, honey, minced garlic, salt, and pepper until evenly coated.

3. Spread Brussels sprouts in a single layer on the prepared baking sheet.

4. Bake in the preheated oven for 25-30 minutes, or until Brussels sprouts are tender and caramelized, stirring halfway through.

5. Remove from the oven and transfer roasted Brussels sprouts to a serving dish.

6. Serve hot, garnished with grated Parmesan cheese and chopped parsley if desired.

- Preparation Time: 10 minutes
- Cooking Time: 25-30 minutes
- Yield: 4 servings
- Nutritional Information (per serving):
- Calories: 120
- Protein: 4g
- Carbohydrates: 15g
- Fat: 6g
- Fiber: 5g

6. Oven-Roasted Cauliflower Steaks

Ingredients:

- 1 large head cauliflower

- 2 tbsp olive oil

- 2 cloves garlic, minced

- 1 tsp smoked paprika

- 1/2 tsp cumin

- Salt and pepper to taste

- Optional garnish: chopped parsley, lemon wedges

Instructions:

1. Preheat the oven to 425°F (220°C). Line a baking sheet with parchment paper.

2. Remove the outer leaves from the cauliflower head and trim the stem, leaving the core intact. Slice cauliflower into 1-inch thick steaks.

3. In a small bowl, whisk together olive oil, minced garlic, smoked paprika, cumin, salt, and pepper.

4. Brush both sides of cauliflower steaks with the olive oil mixture and place them on the prepared baking sheet.

5. Roast in the preheated oven for 20-25 minutes, or until cauliflower is tender and golden brown, flipping halfway through.

6. Remove from the oven and transfer roasted cauliflower steaks to a serving platter.

7. Serve hot, garnished with chopped parsley and lemon wedges if desired.

- - Preparation Time: 10 minutes
- - Cooking Time: 20-25 minutes
- - Yield: 4 servings
- - Nutritional Information (per serving):
- - Calories: 100
- - Protein: 4g
- - Carbohydrates: 10g
- - Fat: 6g
- - Fiber: 4g

7. Honey Glazed Carrots

Ingredients:

- 1 lb carrots, peeled and sliced into rounds

- 2 tbsp olive oil

- 2 tbsp honey

- 1 tbsp balsamic vinegar

- 1 tsp dried thyme

- Salt and pepper to taste

- Optional garnish: chopped parsley

Instructions:

1. Preheat the oven to 400°F (200°C). Line a baking sheet with parchment paper.

2. In a large bowl, toss carrot slices with olive oil, honey, balsamic vinegar, dried thyme, salt, and pepper until evenly coated.

3. Spread carrots in a single layer on the prepared baking sheet.

4. Roast in the preheated oven for 20-25 minutes, or until carrots are tender and caramelized, stirring halfway through.

5. Remove from the oven and transfer roasted carrots to a serving dish.

6. Serve hot, garnished with chopped parsley if desired.

- Preparation Time: 10 minutes
- Cooking Time: 20-25 minutes
- Yield: 4 servings
- Nutritional Information (per serving):

- Calories: 100
- Protein: 1g
- Carbohydrates: 15g
- Fat: 6g
- Fiber: 4g

8. Parmesan Roasted Asparagus

Ingredients:

- 1 lb asparagus spears, trimmed
- 2 tbsp olive oil
- 1/4 cup grated Parmesan cheese
- 2 cloves garlic, minced
- Salt and pepper to taste
- Optional garnish: lemon wedges, chopped parsley

Instructions:

1. Preheat the oven to 425°F (220°C). Line a baking sheet with parchment paper.

2. Place trimmed asparagus spears on the prepared baking sheet.

3. Drizzle olive oil over the asparagus and sprinkle minced garlic, grated Parmesan cheese, salt, and pepper on top.

4. Toss everything together until asparagus spears are evenly coated.

5. Roast in the preheated oven for 12-15 minutes, or until asparagus is tender and Parmesan cheese is golden brown and crispy.

6. Remove from the oven and transfer roasted asparagus to a serving platter.

7. Serve hot, garnished with lemon wedges and chopped parsley if desired.

- Preparation Time: 10 minutes
- Cooking Time: 12-15 minutes
- Yield: 4 servings
- Nutritional Information (per serving):
- Calories: 80
- Protein: 4g
- Carbohydrates: 5g
- Fat: 6g
- Fiber: 3g

Veggie-Forward Casseroles and Grilled Delights

9. Zucchini and Eggplant Lasagna

Ingredients:

- - 2 large zucchini, sliced lengthwise into thin strips
- - 1 large eggplant, sliced lengthwise into thin strips
- - 2 cups marinara sauce
- - 1 cup ricotta cheese
- - 1 cup shredded mozzarella cheese
- - 1/4 cup grated Parmesan cheese
- - 2 cloves garlic, minced
- - 1 tsp dried oregano
- - Salt and pepper to taste
- - Fresh basil leaves for garnish

Instructions:

1. Preheat the oven to 375°F (190°C). Grease a 9x13-inch baking dish with cooking spray.2. In a small bowl, mix together ricotta cheese, minced

garlic, dried oregano, salt, and pepper.

3. Spread a thin layer of marinara sauce on the bottom of the prepared baking dish.

4. Layer zucchini and eggplant slices on top of the marinara sauce, alternating between the two.

5. Spread half of the ricotta mixture over the vegetable layer, followed by half of the remaining marinara sauce.

6. Sprinkle half of the shredded mozzarella cheese and half of the grated Parmesan cheese over the sauce.

7. Repeat the layers with the remaining zucchini, eggplant, ricotta mixture, marinara sauce, shredded mozzarella, and grated Parmesan.

8. Cover the baking dish with aluminum foil and bake in the preheated oven for 30 minutes.

9. Remove the foil and bake for an additional 15-20 minutes, or until the cheese is bubbly and golden brown.

10. Let the lasagna cool for a few minutes before slicing.

11. Serve hot, garnished with fresh basil leaves.

-
- - Preparation Time: 20 minutes
- Cooking Time: 45-55 minutes
- - Yield: 6 servings
- - Nutritional Information (per serving):
- - Calories: 250
- - Protein: 12g
- - Carbohydrates: 15g
- - Fat: 15g
- - Fiber: 5g

10. Grilled Portobello Mushrooms

Ingredients:

- - 4 large portobello mushrooms, stems removed
- - 2 tbsp balsamic vinegar
- - 2 tbsp olive oil
- - 2 cloves garlic, minced
- - 1 tsp dried thyme
- - Salt and pepper to taste

- - Optional garnish: chopped parsley

Instructions:

1. In a shallow dish, whisk together balsamic vinegar, olive oil, minced garlic, dried thyme, salt, and pepper.

2. Add portobello mushrooms to the marinade and toss to coat evenly. Let them marinate for at least 15 minutes.

3. Preheat a grill or grill pan over medium heat. Remove mushrooms from the marinade and shake off any excess.

4. Grill mushrooms for 4-5 minutes on each side, or until they are tender and grill marks appear.

5. Remove from the grill and transfer grilled portobello mushrooms to a serving platter.

6. Serve hot, garnished with chopped parsley if desired.

- Preparation Time: 20 minutes
- Cooking Time: 10 minutes
- Yield: 4 servings

- - Nutritional Information (per serving):
- - Calories: 80
- - Protein: 4g
- - Carbohydrates: 5g
- - Fat: 6g
- - Fiber: 2g

11. Veggie Quinoa Bake

Ingredients:

- - 1 cup quinoa, rinsed and drained
- - 2 cups vegetable broth
- - 2 cups mixed vegetables (such as bell peppers, zucchini, carrots, corn)
- - 1 can (15 oz) black beans, drained and rinsed
- - 1 can (14 oz) diced tomatoes
- - 1 tsp chili powder
- 1/2 tsp cumin
- - Salt and pepper to taste
- - 1 cup shredded cheddar cheese
- - Optional garnish: chopped cilantro, avocado slices

Instructions:

1. Preheat the oven to 375°F (190°C). Grease a 9x13-inch baking dish with cooking spray.

2. In a large saucepan, bring vegetable broth to a boil. Add quinoa, reduce heat to low, cover, and simmer for 15 minutes.

3. In a large bowl, combine cooked quinoa, mixed vegetables, black beans, diced tomatoes, chili powder, cumin, salt, and pepper.

4. Transfer the quinoa mixture to the prepared baking dish and spread it out evenly.

5. Sprinkle shredded cheddar cheese over the top of the quinoa mixture.

6. Cover the baking dish with aluminum foil and bake in the preheated oven for 20 minutes.

- 7. Remove the foil and bake for an additional 10-15 minutes, or until the cheese is melted and bubbly.
- 8. Let the veggie quinoa bake cool for a few minutes before serving.
- 9. Serve hot, garnished with chopped cilantro and avocado slices if desired.
- Preparation Time: 20 minutes
- Cooking Time: 35-40 minutes
- Yield: 6 servings
- Nutritional Information (per serving):
- - Calories: 300
- - Protein: 15g
- - Carbohydrates: 35g
- - Fat: 10g
- - Fiber: 8g
- **12. Stuffed Bell Peppers**
- **Ingredients:**
- - 4 large bell peppers, halved and seeded
- - 1 cup cooked quinoa
- - 1 can (15 oz) black beans, drained and rinsed
- - 1 cup corn kernels
- - 1 cup diced tomatoes
- - 1/2 cup shredded cheddar cheese
- - 2 cloves garlic, minced
- - 1 tsp chili powder
- - 1/2 tsp cumin
- - Salt and pepper to taste

- - Optional garnish: chopped cilantro, sour cream

Instructions:

1. Preheat the oven to 375°F (190°C). Grease a 9x13-inch baking dish with cooking spray.

2. In a large bowl, combine cooked quinoa, black beans, corn kernels, diced tomatoes, shredded cheddar cheese, minced garlic, chili powder, cumin, salt, and pepper.

3. Stuff each bell pepper half with the quinoa mixture and place them in the prepared baking dish.

4. Cover the baking dish with aluminum foil and bake in the preheated oven for 25 minutes.

 5. Remove the foil and bake for an additional 10-15 minutes, or until the peppers are tender.

6. Let the stuffed bell peppers cool for a few minutes before serving.

7. Serve hot, garnished with chopped cilantro and a dollop of sour cream if desired.

- - Preparation Time: 20 minutes
- - Cooking Time: 35-40 minutes
- - Yield: 4 servings
- - Nutritional Information (per serving):
- - Calories: 250
- - Protein: 10g
- - Carbohydrates: 35g
- - Fat: 8g
- - Fiber: 8g

CHAPTER 5

Smart Snacks and Small Bites:

Nutrient-Dense Snack Ideas

1. Almond Butter and Banana Rice Cakes

- **Ingredients:**

  - 4 rice cakes

  - 1/4 cup almond butter

  - 2 bananas, sliced

  - Optional: honey or cinnamon for drizzling

Instructions:

1. Spread almond butter evenly onto each rice cake.

2. Top with banana slices.

3. Drizzle with honey or sprinkle with cinnamon if desired.

4. Serve immediately.

- Preparation Time: 5 minutes
- Yield: 4 servings
- Nutritional Information (per serving):
- Calories: 200
- Protein: 5g
- Carbohydrates: 25g
- Fat: 10g
- Fiber: 3g

2. Veggie Sticks with Hummus

- **Ingredients:**
- 2 large carrots, cut into sticks
- 2 celery stalks, cut into sticks
- 1 cucumber, cut into sticks
- 1 bell pepper, sliced
- 1 cup hummus

Instructions:

1. Arrange veggie sticks on a serving platter.

2. Serve with hummus for dipping

- Preparation Time: 10 minutes
- Yield: 4 servings
- Nutritional Information (per serving):
- Calories: 150
- Protein: 5g
- Carbohydrates: 20g
- Fat: 7g
- Fiber: 7g

3. Greek Yogurt with Honey and Nuts

- Ingredients:

- 2 cups Greek yogurt

- 2 tbsp honey

- 1/4 cup chopped nuts (such as almonds, walnuts, or pecans)

Instructions:

1. Divide Greek yogurt into serving bowls.

2. Drizzle with honey and sprinkle with chopped nuts.

3. Serve immediately.

- - Preparation Time: 5 minutes
- - Yield: 4 servings
- - Nutritional Information (per serving):
- - Calories: 150
- - Protein: 15g
- - Carbohydrates: 10g
- - Fat: 7g
- - Fiber: 1g

4. Cottage Cheese with Pineapple

- Ingredients:

- 2 cups cottage cheese

- 1 cup diced pineapple

Instructions:

1. Divide cottage cheese into serving bowls.

2. Top with diced pineapple.

3. Serve immediately.

- - Preparation Time: 5 minutes
- - Yield: 4 servings
- - Nutritional Information (per serving):
- - Calories: 120
- - Protein: 15g
- - Carbohydrates: 10g
- - Fat: 2g
- - Fiber: 1g
-

5. Trail Mix Energy Balls

Ingredients:

- 1 cup rolled oats

- 1/2 cup nut butter (such as almond or peanut butter)

- 1/4 cup honey

- 1/4 cup chopped nuts

- 1/4 cup dried fruit (such as raisins or cranberries)

- 1/4 cup mini chocolate chips (optional)

Instructions:

1. In a large bowl, combine rolled oats, nut butter, honey, chopped nuts, dried fruit, and mini chocolate chips (if using).

2. Mix until well combined.

3. Roll the mixture into small balls using your hands.

4. Place energy balls on a baking sheet lined with parchment paper.

5. Refrigerate for at least 30 minutes to set.

6. Store in an airtight container in the refrigerator until ready to eat.

- Preparation Time: 15 minutes
- Yield: 12 energy balls
- Nutritional Information (per energy ball):
- Calories: 150
- Protein: 4g
- Carbohydrates: 15g
- Fat: 9g
- Fiber: 2g

6. Turkey and Cheese Roll-Ups

- Ingredients:

- 4 slices turkey breast

- 4 slices cheese (such as cheddar or Swiss)

- Optional: mustard or mayonnaise for spreading

Instructions:

1. Lay a slice of turkey breast flat on a clean surface.

2. Place a slice of cheese on top of the turkey.

3. If desired, spread mustard or mayonnaise on the cheese.

4. Roll up the turkey and cheese tightly.

5. Secure with toothpicks if necessary.

6. Repeat with the remaining turkey and cheese slices.

7. Serve immediately or refrigerate until ready to eat.

- - Preparation Time: 5 minutes
- - Yield: 4 roll-ups
- - Nutritional Information (per roll-up):
- - Calories: 100
- - Protein: 10g
- - Carbohydrates: 1g
- - Fat: 6g
- - Fiber: 0g

7. Apple Slices with Peanut Butter

Ingredients:

- 2 apples, sliced

- 1/4 cup peanut butter

Instructions:

1. Arrange apple slices on a serving plate.

2. Serve with peanut butter for dipping.

- - Preparation Time: 5 minutes
- - Yield: 4 servings
- - Nutritional Information (per serving):
- - Calories: 150
- - Protein: 4g
- - Carbohydrates: 20g
- - Fat: 7g
- - Fiber: 4g

8. Hard-Boiled Eggs

- Ingredients:

- 4 large eggs

Instructions:

1. Place eggs in a single layer in a saucepan.

2. Cover with cold water, making sure the eggs are submerged.

3. Bring water to a boil over medium-high heat.

4. Once boiling, remove the saucepan from heat, cover, and let eggs sit for 10-12 minutes.

5. Transfer eggs to a bowl of ice water and let cool for a few minutes.

6. Peel eggs and serve immediately or refrigerate until ready to eat.

- - Preparation Time: 5 minutes
- - Cooking Time: 12 minutes
- - Yield: 4 servings
- - Nutritional Information (per serving):
- - Calories: 70
- - Protein: 6g
- - Carbohydrates: 0g
- - Fat: 5g
- - Fiber: 0g

CHAPTER 6

Delectable Desserts
Guilt-Free Sweet Treats

1. Dark Chocolate Avocado Mousse

Ingredients:

- 2 ripe avocados, peeled and pitted

- 1/4 cup unsweetened cocoa powder

- 1/4 cup maple syrup or honey

- 1/4 cup almond milk

- 1 tsp vanilla extract

- Pinch of salt

- Optional toppings: fresh berries, shaved dark chocolate

Instructions:

1. In a food processor or blender, combine avocados, cocoa powder, maple syrup or honey, almond milk, vanilla extract, and salt.

2. Blend until smooth and creamy, scraping down the sides as needed.

3. Transfer the mousse to serving dishes and chill in the refrigerator for at least 30 minutes.

4. Serve cold, topped with fresh berries and shaved dark chocolate if desired.

- - Preparation Time: 10 minutes
- - Chill Time: 30 minutes
- - Yield: 4 servings
- - Nutritional Information (per serving):
- - Calories: 200
- - Protein: 3g
- - Carbohydrates: 20g
- - Fat: 15g
- - Fiber: 6g

2. Berry Frozen Yogurt Bites

Ingredients:

- 1 cup Greek yogurt

- 1 cup mixed berries (such as strawberries, blueberries, raspberries)

- 1 tbsp honey (optional)

Instructions:

1. In a bowl, mix Greek yogurt with honey (if using) until smooth.

2. Line a mini muffin tin with paper liners.

3. Spoon a small amount of yogurt into each muffin cup, filling them halfway.

4. Place a few mixed berries on top of the yogurt in each cup.

5. Top with the remaining yogurt, covering the berries.

6. Freeze for at least 2 hours, or until firm.

7. Remove from the muffin tin and peel off the paper liners before serving.

- - Preparation Time: 10 minutes
- - Freezing Time: 2 hours
- - Yield: 12 yogurt bites
- - Nutritional Information (per yogurt bite):
- - Calories: 30
- - Protein: 2g
- - Carbohydrates: 4g
- - Fat: 0g
- - Fiber: 1g

3. Banana Nice Cream

Ingredients:

- 2 ripe bananas, peeled and sliced

- 1/4 cup almond milk

- 1 tsp vanilla extract

- Optional toppings: sliced bananas, chopped nuts, dark chocolate chips

Instructions:

1. Place sliced bananas in a single layer on a baking sheet lined with parchment paper.

2. Freeze for at least 2 hours, or until solid.

3. In a blender or food processor, combine frozen bananas, almond milk, and vanilla extract.

4. Blend until smooth and creamy, scraping down the sides as needed.

5. Transfer the nice cream to serving bowls and top with your favorite toppings.

- 6. Serve immediately.
- - Preparation Time: 5 minutes
- - Freezing Time: 2 hours
- - Yield: 2 servings
- - Nutritional Information (per serving):
- - Calories: 100
- - Protein: 1g
- - Carbohydrates: 25g
- - Fat: 0g
- - Fiber: 3g

4. Chia Seed Pudding with Berries

Ingredients:

- 1/4 cup chia seeds

- 1 cup almond milk

- 1 tbsp maple syrup or honey

- 1/2 tsp vanilla extract

- 1 cup mixed berries (such as strawberries, blueberries, raspberries)

Instructions:

1. In a bowl, whisk together chia seeds, almond milk, maple syrup or honey, and vanilla extract.

2. Cover and refrigerate for at least 2 hours, or overnight, until thickened.

3. Stir the chia pudding to redistribute the seeds.

4. Divide the pudding into serving glasses or bowls.

5. Top with mixed berries before serving.

- - Preparation Time: 5 minutes
- - Chill Time: 2 hours
- - Yield: 2 servings
- - Nutritional Information (per serving):
- - Calories: 150
- - Protein: 4g
- - Carbohydrates: 20g
- - Fat: 7g
- - Fiber: 10g
-

5. Grilled Pineapple with Honey Drizzle

Ingredients:

- 1 pineapple, peeled, cored, and sliced into rings

- 2 tbsp honey

- Optional: vanilla ice cream or Greek yogurt for serving

Instructions:

1. Preheat the grill or grill pan to medium-high heat.

2. Grill pineapple slices for 2-3 minutes on each side, or until grill marks appear and pineapple is slightly caramelized.

3. Drizzle grilled pineapple with honey.

4. Serve hot, with a scoop of vanilla ice cream or Greek yogurt if desired.

- - Preparation Time: 10 minutes
- - Cooking Time: 6 minutes
- - Yield: 4 servings

- - Nutritional Information (per serving, without ice cream or yogurt):
- - Calories: 100
- - Protein: 1g
- - Carbohydrates: 25g
- - Fat: 0g
- - Fiber: 2g

6. Mixed Berry Crisp

Ingredients:

- 4 cups mixed berries (such as strawberries, blueberries, raspberries)

- 1 tbsp lemon juice

- 1/4 cup maple syrup or honey

- 1/2 cup rolled oats

- 1/4 cup almond flour

- 2 tbsp coconut oil, melted

- 1/4 tsp cinnamon

- Pinch of salt

Instructions:

1. Preheat the oven to 375°F (190°C). Grease a baking dish with coconut oil.

2. In a large bowl, toss mixed berries with lemon juice and maple syrup or honey. Transfer to the prepared baking dish.

3. In the same bowl, combine rolled oats, almond flour, melted coconut oil, cinnamon, and salt.

4. Sprinkle the oat mixture over the berries in the baking dish.

5. Bake in the preheated oven for 25-30 minutes, or until the topping is golden brown and the berries are bubbling.

6. Remove from the oven and let cool for a few minutes before serving.

7. Serve warm, optionally with a scoop of vanilla ice cream or Greek yogurt.

- - Preparation Time: 15 minutes
- - Cooking Time: 25-30 minutes
- - Yield: 6 servings

- - Nutritional Information (per serving, without ice cream or yogurt):
- - Calories: 180
- - Protein: 3g
- - Carbohydrates: 30g
- - Fat: 7g
- - Fiber: 5g

7. Peach and Mango Sorbet

Ingredients:

- 2 ripe peaches, peeled and diced

- 1 ripe mango, peeled and diced

- 1/4 cup honey or maple syrup

- 1 tbsp lemon juice

Instructions:

1. Place diced peaches and mango in a blender or food processor.

2. Add honey or maple syrup and lemon juice.

3. Blend until smooth.

4. Transfer the mixture to a shallow dish or baking pan.

5. Freeze for at least 4 hours, or until firm.

6. Once frozen, use a fork to scrape the sorbet to create a slushy texture.

7. Serve immediately or transfer to an airtight container and store in the freezer.

- - Preparation Time: 10 minutes
- - Freezing Time: 4 hours
- - Yield: 4 servings
- - Nutritional Information (per serving):
- - Calories: 100
- - Protein: 1g
- - Carbohydrates: 25g
- - Fat: 0g
- - Fiber: 2g

8. Fruit Salad with Honey Lime Dressing

Ingredients:

- 2 cups mixed fruit (such as strawberries, blueberries, kiwi, pineapple, grapes)

- 2 tbsp honey

- 1 tbsp lime juice

- Zest of 1 lime

- Optional: fresh mint leaves for garnish

Instructions:

1. In a large bowl, combine mixed fruit.

2. In a small bowl, whisk together honey, lime juice, and lime zest.

3. Pour the dressing over the fruit and toss gently to coat.

4. Garnish with fresh mint leaves if desired.

5. Serve immediately or refrigerate until ready to eat.

- - Preparation Time: 10 minutes
- - Yield: 4 servings
- - Nutritional Information (per serving):
- - Calories: 70
- - Protein: 1g
- - Carbohydrates: 18g
- - Fat: 0g
- - Fiber: 2g

CHAPTER 7

Hydration and Beverage
Infused Water Creations

1. Cucumber Mint Infused Water

Ingredients:

- 1/2 cucumber, thinly sliced

- 10 fresh mint leaves

- 4 cups water

- Ice cubes (optional)

Instructions:

1. In a pitcher, combine cucumber slices and mint leaves.

2. Fill the pitcher with water.

3. Refrigerate for at least 2 hours, or overnight, to allow the flavors to infuse.

4. Serve chilled, with ice cubes if desired.

- - Preparation Time: 5 minutes
- - Infusion Time: 2 hours
- - Yield: 4 servings
- - Nutritional Information (per serving):
- - Calories: 0
- - Protein: 0g
- - Carbohydrates: 0g
- - Fat: 0g
- - Fiber: 0g

2. Citrus Berry Infused Water

Ingredients:

- 1/2 cup mixed berries (such as strawberries, blueberries, raspberries)

- 1 orange, thinly sliced

- 4 cups water

- Ice cubes (optional)

Instructions:

1. In a pitcher, combine mixed berries and orange slices.

2. Fill the pitcher with water.

3. Refrigerate for at least 2 hours, or overnight, to allow the flavors to infuse.

4. Serve chilled, with ice cubes if desired.

- - Preparation Time: 5 minutes
- - Infusion Time: 2 hours
- - Yield: 4 servings
- - Nutritional Information (per serving):

- - Calories: 10
- - Protein: 0g
- - Carbohydrates: 3g
- - Fat: 0g
- - Fiber: 1g

Protein-Packed Smoothie Recipes

3. Green Protein Power Smoothie

Ingredients:

- - 1 cup spinach
- - 1/2 banana
- - 1/2 cup Greek yogurt
- - 1/2 cup almond milk
- - 1 scoop vanilla protein powder
- - Optional: honey or maple syrup for sweetness
- - Ice cubes (optional)

Instructions:

1. In a blender, combine spinach, banana, Greek yogurt, almond milk, and protein powder.

2. Blend until smooth and creamy.

3. Taste and add honey or maple syrup for sweetness if desired.

4. Add ice cubes and blend again until smooth.

5. Serve immediately.

- - Preparation Time: 5 minutes
- - Yield: 1 serving
- - Nutritional Information (per serving):
- - Calories: 250
- - Protein: 25g
- - Carbohydrates: 25g
- - Fat: 5g
- - Fiber: 5g
-

4. Berry Blast Smoothie

Ingredients:

- 1/2 cup mixed berries (such as strawberries, blueberries, raspberries)

- 1/2 banana

- 1/2 cup Greek yogurt

- 1/2 cup almond milk

- 1 scoop vanilla protein powder

- Optional: honey or maple syrup for sweetness

- Ice cubes (optional)

Instructions:

1. In a blender, combine mixed berries, banana, Greek yogurt, almond milk, and protein powder.

2. Blend until smooth and creamy.

3. Taste and add honey or maple syrup for sweetness if desired.

4. Add ice cubes and blend again until smooth.

5. Serve immediately.

- - Preparation Time: 5 minutes
- - Yield: 1 serving
- - Nutritional Information (per serving):
- - Calories: 250
- - Protein: 25g
- - Carbohydrates: 25g
- - Fat: 5g
- - Fiber: 5g
-

Herbal Teas and Other Hydration Tips

5. Ginger Turmeric Tea

Ingredients:

- 2 cups water

- 1-inch piece of ginger, peeled and thinly sliced

- 1-inch piece of turmeric, peeled and thinly sliced

- Honey to taste

Instructions:

1. In a saucepan, bring water to a boil.

2. Add ginger and turmeric slices to the boiling water.

3. Reduce heat and let simmer for 10-15 minutes.

4. Strain the tea into mugs and sweeten with honey to taste.

5. Serve hot.

- Preparation Time: 5 minutes
- - Cooking Time: 15 minutes
- - Yield: 2 servings

- - Nutritional Information (per serving):
- - Calories: 10
- - Protein: 0g
- - Carbohydrates: 3g
- - Fat: 0g
- - Fiber: 0g

6. Hibiscus Iced Tea

Ingredients:

- 4 cups water

- 2 hibiscus tea bags

- 2 tbsp honey or maple syrup (optional)

- Ice cubes

- Lemon slices for garnish (optional)

Instructions:

1. Bring water to a boil in a saucepan.

2. Remove from heat and add hibiscus tea bags.

3. Let steep for 5-10 minutes, depending on desired strength.

4. Remove tea bags and stir in honey or maple syrup if using.

5. Allow the tea to cool to room temperature, then transfer to a pitcher and refrigerate until cold.

6. Serve over ice cubes, garnished with lemon slices if desired.

- - Preparation Time: 5 minutes
- - Cooking Time: 5-10 minutes
- - Chill Time: 1-2 hours
- - Yield: 4 servings
- - Nutritional Information (per serving):
- - Calories: 10
- - Protein: 0g
- - Carbohydrates: 3g
- - Fat: 0g
- - Fiber: 0g

CHAPTER 8

Meal Planning and Preparation Strategies

Meal planning and preparation are critical components of leading a healthy lifestyle, especially for those who have had gastric sleeve surgery. These measures not only assure a well-balanced diet, but also aid with portion control and lowering the danger of overeating. In this thorough book, we will dig into the complexities of meal planning, batch cooking, freezing ideas, and eating out methods to provide you with the knowledge and skills you need to succeed on your weight loss journey after surgery.

Weekly Meal Planning Guidelines

A weekly meal plan serves as a guide for your dietary choices throughout the week. It helps you plan your meals, provides balanced nutrition, and reduces the temptation to eat bad foods. Here's a step-by-step method for creating an effective weekly food plan.

1. Determine Your Nutritional Needs: Begin by determining your unique nutritional needs, taking into account protein intake, fiber consumption, and vital vitamins and minerals. Consult a licensed dietitian or nutritionist to create individualized dietary advice based on your individual needs and interests.

2. Plan Balanced Meals: Try to include a range of dietary categories at each meal, such as lean proteins, healthy fats, complex carbs, and a rainbow of colorful fruits and vegetables. Strive for balance and diversity in your meals to ensure they are both nutritious and delicious.

3. Choose Gastric Sleeve-Friendly Recipes. Choose recipes created exclusively for those who have had gastric sleeve surgery. These recipes

often stress lower portion sizes, high protein content, and nutrient-dense foods to aid with weight reduction and satiety.

4. Create a Grocery List: Once you've chosen your dishes for the week, make a detailed grocery list that includes all of the products you'll need. Organize your list by food category to make shopping easier and prevent you from missing any crucial products.

5. Schedule Meal Preparation Time: Set aside a set day or time each week for meal prep and batch cooking. This lets you to easily cut vegetables, marinade meats, and prepare freezer-friendly meals ahead of time, saving you time and effort on hectic weekdays.

6. Maintain Flexibility: While having a meal plan is essential, it is also critical to remain flexible and adaptable. Life frequently brings unexpected changes and challenges, so be prepared to modify your meal plan as necessary. Keep a collection of quick and easy recipes on hand for hectic days or unexpected events.

7. Reflect and Revise: At the conclusion of each week, spend some time to review your meal plan and determine what went well and what may be improved. Use this input to improve your meal planning process and make changes as needed to better suit your nutritional goals and lifestyle.

By following these principles, you may develop a personalized weekly meal plan that meets your nutritional needs, aids in weight reduction, and promotes overall health and well-being.

Tips for Batch Cooking and Freezing.

Batch cooking and freezing are excellent solutions for saving time, reducing food waste, and ensuring that you always have healthful meals on hand. Here are some recommendations for increasing the efficiency and efficacy of batch cooking and freezing:

1. Select Freezer-Friendly Recipes. Choose freezer-friendly recipes, such as soups, stews, casseroles, and protein-based dishes. These meals frequently keep their flavor and texture when frozen and reheated.

2. Invest in Quality Storage Containers: To keep your frozen meals fresh, use high-quality freezer-safe containers and storage bags. Choose containers with tight-sealing lids to avoid freezer burn and preserve freshness.

3. Label and Date Everything: Clearly label your freezer dinners with the recipe name and date of preparation. This makes it easy to recognize and track your

meals' freshness, allowing you to eat them before they expire.

4. Practice Portion Control: To prevent overeating, divide your batch-cooked meals into individual or family-sized servings. To prepare meals ahead of time, consider utilizing portion-controlled containers or silicone muffin cups.

5. Use Freezer-Friendly Ingredients. Incorporate freezer-friendly components into your batch-made meals, such as prepared grains, beans, diced veggies, and pre-cooked meats like chicken, turkey, or lean beef. These items are readily incorporated into a number of dishes to provide quick and simple dinners.

6. Rotate Your Freezer Stock: Rotate your freezer stock on a regular basis to ensure that older foods are used first, reducing food waste and providing a fresh supply of

meals at all times. To prioritize older products, organize your freezer according to the first-in, first-out (FIFO) principle.

7. defrost Safely: To avoid foodborne disease, defrost frozen meals properly. Thaw meals in the refrigerator overnight, or use your microwave's defrost mode for faster thawing. Avoid thawing at room temperature, as this can encourage bacterial growth.

By implementing these batch cooking and freezing strategies into your meal planning routine, you can streamline your food preparation process, reduce cooking time on hectic weekdays, and enjoy the convenience of having healthy meals on hand whenever you need them.

Dining Out Strategies for Success

Dining out can pose challenges for individuals following a gastric sleeve surgery diet, but with careful planning and mindful choices, it's possible to enjoy restaurant meals while staying on track with your health and weight loss goals. Here are some strategies for dining out success:

1. Research Restaurants in Advance: Before dining out, review restaurant menus online to identify options that align with your dietary preferences and nutritional goals. Look for restaurants that offer a variety of protein-rich dishes, salads, and vegetable sides to accommodate your needs.

2. Practice Portion Control: Restaurant portions are often larger than what you would typically consume at home, making portion control essential. Consider sharing entrees with a

dining companion, ordering appetizer-sized portions, or asking for a to-go box to portion out half of your meal before you begin eating.

3. Prioritize Protein: Protein is crucial for supporting muscle repair, promoting satiety, and aiding in weight loss. Choose protein-rich options such as grilled chicken, fish, lean beef, or tofu as the focal point of your meal, and pair them with vegetable sides or salads for a well-balanced plate.

4.Request Modifications: Don't hesitate to request modifications to menu items to better suit your dietary needs. Ask for grilled or baked preparations instead of fried, request dressings and sauces on the side, and substitute high-calorie sides with steamed vegetables or a side salad to reduce calorie intake and improve nutritional value.

5. Practice Mindful Eating: Adopt mindful eating practices when dining out by paying attention to hunger and fullness cues, eating slowly, and savoring each bite. Put your fork down between bites, take small sips of water, and engage in conversation to prolong your mealtime experience and prevent overeating.

6. Be Mindful of Liquid Calories: Be cautious of liquid calories from beverages such as sugary cocktails, sodas, and sweetened iced teas, as they can contribute to excess calorie intake. Opt for calorie-free options like water, unsweetened tea, or sparkling water with a splash of lemon or lime to stay hydrated without adding extra calories.

7. Plan Ahead for Special Occasions: If you have a special occasion or dining event planned, anticipate the menu offerings in advance and plan your choices accordingly. Consider eating a small,

protein-rich snack before you go to help curb your appetite and prevent overindulgence. Look for healthier options on the menu, and don't be afraid to ask for modifications to better align with your dietary goals.

By implementing these dining out strategies, you can navigate restaurant menus with confidence, make informed choices that support your health and weight loss goals, and enjoy dining out as a pleasurable and social experience without derailing your progress.

In conclusion, meal planning and preparation are essential components of a successful post-gastric sleeve surgery lifestyle. By incorporating weekly meal planning guides, batch cooking and freezing tips, and dining out strategies for success, you can effectively manage your dietary intake, make healthy choices, and achieve long-term success on your weight loss journey. These strategies empower you to take control of your nutrition, support your overall health and well-being, and maintain a balanced and sustainable approach to eating for years to come. Remember that consistency, mindfulness, and flexibility are key to navigating the challenges and opportunities that arise on your path to health and wellness. With dedication and perseverance, you can create a fulfilling and nourishing relationship with food that enhances your quality of life and helps you achieve your desired health outcomes.

Maintaining Motivation and Lifestyle Changes

Embarking on a journey towards a healthier lifestyle, especially after undergoing gastric sleeve surgery, requires not only determination but also sustained motivation and commitment. In this comprehensive guide, we will explore various aspects of maintaining motivation and making lasting lifestyle changes, including setting realistic goals, overcoming challenges and plateaus, and celebrating successes along the way. By understanding these key elements and incorporating them into your daily routine, you can stay motivated and resilient on your path to long-term health and well-being.

Setting Realistic Goals

Setting realistic goals is essential for maintaining motivation and sustaining progress over time. Here's how to set achievable goals that will keep you motivated on your journey:

1. Be Specific: Define your goals with clarity and specificity. Instead of setting vague goals like "lose weight," specify how much weight you want to lose and by when. For example, "lose 10 pounds in three months."

2. Make Them Measurable: Ensure that your goals are measurable so that you can track your progress and celebrate your achievements along the way. Use metrics such as pounds lost, inches dropped, or changes in body composition to measure your success.

3. Set Short-Term and Long-Term Goals: Break down your larger, long-term goals into smaller, manageable short-term goals. This makes your objectives more achievable and allows you to experience a sense of accomplishment more frequently, keeping you motivated to continue working towards your ultimate goal.

4. Be Realistic: Set goals that are challenging yet attainable based on your current circumstances, capabilities, and resources. Avoid setting unrealistic goals that may set you up for disappointment and frustration.

5. Focus on Behavior Changes: Instead of solely focusing on outcomes like weight loss, shift your focus to behavior changes that support your goals. For example, set goals related to dietary changes, physical activity, hydration, and stress management.

6. Write Them Down: Document your goals in writing and review them regularly to keep them top of mind. Consider creating a vision board or using a goal-tracking app to visually represent your goals and progress.

7. Adjust as Needed: Be flexible and willing to adjust your goals as needed based on your evolving circumstances, preferences, and priorities. Celebrate your achievements, no matter how small, and use setbacks as opportunities to learn and grow.

By setting realistic and achievable goals, you can maintain motivation and stay focused on making meaningful progress towards your health and wellness objectives.

Overcoming Challenges and Plateaus

On the journey towards improved health and well-being, it's inevitable to encounter challenges and plateaus along the way. Here's how to navigate these obstacles and stay resilient in the face of adversity:

1. Anticipate Challenges: Identify potential obstacles that may arise on your journey, such as cravings, social pressure, emotional eating, or time constraints. By anticipating these challenges, you can proactively develop strategies to overcome them when they occur.

2. Seek Support: Don't hesitate to reach out for support from

friends, family members, support groups, or healthcare professionals when facing challenges. Having a strong support network can provide encouragement, accountability, and practical guidance to help you overcome obstacles and stay on track.

3. Practice Self-Compassion: Be kind to yourself and practice self-compassion during challenging times. Acknowledge that setbacks are a natural part of the process and treat yourself with the same kindness and understanding that you would offer to a friend facing similar struggles.

4. Focus on Progress, Not Perfection: Instead of striving for perfection, focus on progress and celebrate the small victories along the way. Recognize that progress is not always linear and that even small steps forward are significant achievements worthy of celebration.

5. Reassess Your Approach: If you find yourself stuck in a plateau or facing recurring challenges, take a step back and reassess your approach. Evaluate your behaviors, habits, and strategies to identify areas for improvement and make necessary adjustments to your plan.

6. Stay Patient and Persistent: Stay patient and persistent, even when progress seems slow or obstacles seem insurmountable. Remember that meaningful change takes time, and consistency is key to long-term success.

7. Focus on Non-Scale Victories: Don't solely rely on the scale to measure your progress. Celebrate non-scale victories such as improved energy levels, better sleep, increased strength and endurance, and positive changes in mood and mindset.

By adopting a proactive mindset, seeking support when needed, and staying resilient in the face of challenges and plateaus, you can overcome obstacles and continue moving forward on your journey towards improved health and well-being.

Celebrating Successes Along the Way

Celebrating successes, no matter how small, is essential for maintaining motivation and reinforcing positive behaviors. Here are some meaningful ways to celebrate your achievements along the way:

1. Acknowledge Your Progress: Take time to acknowledge and celebrate your progress, no matter how small. Recognize the effort and dedication you've put into making positive changes in your life and give yourself credit for your accomplishments.

2. Set Milestone Rewards: Establish milestone rewards for reaching specific goals or milestones along your journey. Choose rewards that are meaningful to you and alignwith your health and wellness goals, such as treating yourself to a massage, buying a new workout outfit, or enjoying a relaxing day at the spa.

3. Share Your Successes: Share your successes with friends, family, or members of a support group who can offer encouragement and celebrate your achievements with you. Celebrating your victories with others can amplify the joy and motivation you feel and strengthen your support network.

4. Create a Celebration Ritual: Develop a personal celebration ritual that you can use to mark your achievements. This could involve lighting a candle, writing in a journal, or taking a moment of gratitude to reflect on your

progress and express appreciation for your efforts.

5. Document Your Journey: Keep a journal or create a visual progress chart to document your journey and track your successes over time. Celebrate milestones by revisiting your journal entries or progress photos and reflecting on how far you've come since you started.

6. Celebrate Non-Scale Victories: Don't limit your celebrations to scale victories alone. Celebrate non-scale victories such as improved energy levels, better sleep, increased strength and flexibility, and enhanced mood and confidence. These achievements are just as important and worthy of celebration as changes in weight or body composition.

7. Practice Gratitude: Cultivate an attitude of gratitude by expressing appreciation for the progress you've made and the positive changes in your life. Take time each day to acknowledge the things you're grateful for, whether it's improved health, supportive relationships, or newfound confidence and self-esteem.

8. Pay It Forward: Pay it forward by using your success as inspiration to motivate and support others on their own health and wellness journeys. Share your experiences, offer encouragement, and celebrate the successes of others, creating a ripple effect of positivity and empowerment.

By celebrating your successes along the way, you reinforce positive behaviors, boost your confidence and self-esteem, and cultivate a sense of accomplishment and pride in your achievements. Remember that every step forward, no matter how small, is a cause for celebration and an opportunity to reaffirm your commitment to your health and well-being.

In conclusion, maintaining motivation and making lasting lifestyle changes after gastric sleeve surgery require dedication, perseverance, and a supportive environment. By setting realistic goals, overcoming challenges and plateaus, and celebrating successes along the way, you can stay motivated, resilient, and empowered on your journey towards improved health and wellness. Embrace the journey, celebrate your victories, and continue striving towards becoming the healthiest and happiest version of yourself. With determination and support, you can achieve your goals and create a fulfilling and vibrant life beyond surgery.

CHAPTER 9

Resources and Support

Embarking on a journey towards improved health and well-being, especially after undergoing gastric sleeve surgery, can be both exhilarating and challenging. Having access to the right resources and support systems can significantly impact an individual's success and resilience throughout this journey. In this comprehensive guide, we will delve into the importance of support groups and communities, as well as provide additional tips and advice for long-term success after gastric sleeve surgery.

Support Groups and Communities

Support groups and communities serve as pillars of strength, encouragement, and guidance for individuals navigating the complexities of life post-gastric sleeve surgery. These groups, whether in-person or online, offer a nurturing environment where individuals can share their experiences, seek advice, and find solace in the company of others who understand their journey. Here are some key reasons why support groups and communities are invaluable resources for long-term success:

1. Emotional Support: Adjusting to life after gastric sleeve surgery can evoke a myriad of

emotions, ranging from elation and empowerment to anxiety and uncertainty. Support groups provide a safe space where individuals can express their feelings openly and receive empathy, validation, and encouragement from fellow members who share similar experiences.

2. Practical Guidance: Support groups offer a wealth of practical advice, tips, and strategies for navigating the post-surgery landscape. Members share insights on topics such as meal planning, nutrition, exercise, managing cravings, and coping with challenges, drawing from their own successes and setbacks to provide valuable guidance to others.

3. Accountability and Motivation: Being part of a support group fosters a sense of accountability and motivation to stay committed to one's health and wellness goals. Sharing progress, setbacks, and successes with peers creates a supportive accountability system that encourages individuals to stay on track, even when faced with obstacles.

4. Community Connection: Support groups cultivate a sense of belonging and camaraderie among members who share a common goal of improving their health and quality of life. Building relationships with like-minded individuals who understand the triumphs and tribulations of the weight loss journey reduces feelings of

isolation and fosters a sense of community and solidarity.

5. Education and Empowerment: Support groups offer opportunities for education and empowerment through guest speakers, workshops, and educational materials. Topics may include nutrition, exercise physiology, mindfulness, body image, and self-care, empowering members with knowledge and tools to make informed decisions about their health and well-being.

6. Celebration of Milestones: Support groups celebrate milestones, both big and small, along the weight loss journey. Whether it's reaching a certain weight loss goal, adopting a new healthy habit, or achieving a non-scale victory, members cheer each other on and celebrate successes together, reinforcing positive behaviors and boosting morale.

7. Long-Term Relationships: Support groups often foster long-term relationships and friendships that extend beyond the confines of the group meetings or online forums. These relationships provide ongoing encouragement, inspiration, and support, creating a sense of community that endures long after reaching weight loss goals.

Additional Tips and Advice for Long-Term Success

In addition to the support provided by support groups and communities, there are several additional tips and strategies that can contribute to long-term success after gastric sleeve surgery:

1. Commit to Lifelong Healthy Habits: Recognize that gastric sleeve surgery is a tool to aid weight loss, but long-term success depends on adopting and maintaining healthy lifestyle habits. Commit to making permanent changes to your diet, exercise, and self-care routines to support your overall health and well-being.

2. Stay Consistent with Follow-Up Care: Attend all scheduled follow-up appointments with your healthcare team, including your surgeon, dietitian, and other specialists. These appointments allow for ongoing monitoring of your progress, adjustments to your treatment plan as needed,

and support for any challenges or concerns that arise.

3. Prioritize Protein and Nutrient-Rich Foods: Protein is essential for supporting muscle repair, promoting satiety, and preventing muscle loss after surgery. Make protein-rich foods a priority in your diet, such as lean meats, poultry, fish, eggs, dairy products, tofu, legumes, and protein supplements recommended by your healthcare team.

4. Stay Hydrated: Adequate hydration is essential for overall health and well-being, especially after gastric sleeve surgery. Aim to drink at least 64 ounces of water per day, sipping slowly throughout the day to avoid dehydration. Avoid calorie-laden beverages such as sugary sodas, juices, and energy drinks, as

they can contribute to excess calorie intake and hinder weight loss efforts.

5. Practice Mindful Eating: Adopt mindful eating practices to enhance awareness of hunger and fullness cues, improve digestion, and prevent overeating. Eat slowly, chew food thoroughly, savor each bite, and pay attention to physical hunger and satiety signals to avoid mindless eating and promote mindful food choices.

6. Incorporate Physical Activity: Engage in regular physical activity to support weight loss, improve cardiovascular health, boost mood, and enhance overall well-being. Aim for a combination of aerobic exercise, strength training, and flexibility exercises to achieve optimal fitness and health benefits. Start slowly and gradually increase the intensity and duration of your workouts as your fitness level improves.

7. Practice Self-Care: Prioritize self-care activities that promote relaxation, stress reduction, and emotional well-being. Practice mindfulness meditation, yoga, deep breathing exercises, journaling, spending time in nature, or engaging in hobbies and activities that bring you joy and fulfillment.

8. Seek Professional Support: If you're struggling with mental health issues, body image concerns, disordered eating behaviors, or other challenges, don't hesitate to seek professional support from a therapist, counselor, or mental

health professional. Addressing these issues early can prevent them from interfering with your long-term success and overall quality of life.

Incorporating these additional tips and strategies into your post-surgery routine can enhance your chances of long-term success and support your ongoing health and wellness goals. Remember that every small step you take towards adopting healthier habits and prioritizing self-care contributes to your overall well-being and enhances your quality of life in meaningful ways.

In conclusion, finding the right resources and support systems, such as support groups and communities, is essential for long-term success after gastric sleeve surgery. By connecting with others who understand your journey, sharing experiences, and accessing valuable information and guidance, you can stay motivated, empowered, and resilient on your path to improved health and well-being. Additionally, incorporating additional tips and strategies for long-term success into your daily routine can further support your ongoing progress and help you achieve your health and wellness goals. Remember that you're not alone on this journey, and with the right support, guidance, and determination, you can create a healthier, happier, and more fulfilling life beyond surgery.

30 DAYS MEAL PLAN

Week 1:

Day 1:

- Breakfast: Spinach and Feta Omelette

- Snack: Almond Butter and Banana Rice Cakes

- Lunch: Grilled Chicken Caesar Salad

- Snack: Greek Yogurt with Honey and Nuts

- Dinner: Lemon Herb Roast Chicken with Roasted Vegetables

Day 2:

- Breakfast: Greek Yogurt Parfait with Berries

- Snack: Mixed Nuts

- Lunch: Butternut Squash Soup with a Side Salad

- Snack: Veggie Sticks with Hummus

- Dinner: Teriyaki Tofu Stir-Fry

Day 3:

- Breakfast: Avocado Toast with Poached Egg

- Snack: Cottage Cheese with Pineapple

- Lunch: Lentil Soup with Whole Grain Bread

- Snack: Trail Mix Energy Balls

- Dinner: Baked Salmon with Dill Sauce and Steamed Broccoli

Day 4:

- Breakfast: Overnight Oats with Chia Seeds

- Snack: Apple Slices with Peanut Butter

- Lunch: Thai Beef Salad

- Snack: Turkey and Cheese Roll-Ups

- Dinner: Turkey and Veggie Meatballs with Zucchini Noodles

Day 5:

- Breakfast: Breakfast Egg Muffins

- Snack: Carrot Sticks with Hummus

- Lunch: Caprese Salad

- Snack: Hard-Boiled Eggs

- Dinner: Chicken Stir-Fry with Veggies

Day 6:

- Breakfast: Dark Chocolate Avocado Mousse

- Snack: Berry Frozen Yogurt Bites

- Lunch: Grilled Chicken Caesar Salad

- Snack: Greek Yogurt Parfait with Berries

- Dinner: Chicken and Broccoli Casserole

Day 7:

- Breakfast: Mixed Berry Crisp

- Snack: Turkey and Cheese Roll-Ups

- Lunch: Lentil Soup with a Side of Steamed Green Beans

- Snack: Almond Butter and Banana Rice Cakes

- Dinner: Shrimp and Veggie Stir-Fry

Week 2:

Day 8:

- Breakfast: Spinach and Feta Omelette

- Snack: Cottage Cheese with Pineapple

- Lunch: Mediterranean Quinoa Salad

- Snack: Veggie Sticks with Hummus

- Dinner: Grilled Chicken Skewers with Peanut Sauce

Day 9:

- Breakfast: Greek Yogurt Parfait with Berries

- Snack: Mixed Nuts

- Lunch: Creamy Tomato Basil Soup with a Side Salad

- Snack: Greek Yogurt with Honey and Nuts

- Dinner: Garlic Butter Grilled Shrimp with Roasted Asparagus

Day 10:

- Breakfast: Avocado Toast with Poached Egg

- Snack: Apple Slices with Peanut Butter

- Lunch: Chicken and Vegetable Soup

- Snack: Trail Mix Energy Balls

- Dinner: Lemon Herb Baked Cod with Steamed Broccoli

Day 11:

- Breakfast: Overnight Oats with Chia Seeds

- Snack: Carrot Sticks with Hummus

- Lunch: Thai Beef Salad

- Snack: Hard-Boiled Eggs

- Dinner: Beef and Veggie Stir-Fry

Day 12:

- Breakfast: Breakfast Egg Muffins

- Snack: Almond Butter and Banana Rice Cakes

- Lunch: Grilled Chicken Caesar Salad

- Snack: Cottage Cheese with Pineapple

- Dinner: Pork Tenderloin with Apple Chutney and Honey Glazed Carrots

Day 13:

- Breakfast: Dark Chocolate Avocado Mousse

- Snack: Berry Frozen Yogurt Bites

- Lunch: Lentil Soup with Whole Grain Bread

- Snack: Greek Yogurt with Honey and Nuts

- Dinner: Turkey Chili

Day 14:

- Breakfast: Mixed Berry Crisp

- Snack: Veggie Sticks with Hummus

- Lunch: Caprese Salad

- Snack: Apple Slices with Peanut Butter

- Dinner: Chicken and Broccoli Casserole

Week 3:

Day 15:

- Breakfast: Spinach and Feta Omelette

- Snack: Mixed Nuts

- Lunch: Grilled Chicken Caesar Salad

- Snack: Greek Yogurt with Honey and Nuts

- Dinner: Grilled Portobello Mushrooms with Steamed Broccoli

Day 16:

- Breakfast: Greek Yogurt Parfait with Berries

- Snack: Cottage Cheese with Pineapple

- Lunch: Butternut Squash Soup with a Side Salad

- Snack: Turkey and Cheese Roll-Ups

- Dinner: Teriyaki Tofu Stir-Fry

Day 17:

- Breakfast: Avocado Toast with Poached Egg

- Snack: Carrot Sticks with Hummus

- Lunch: Chicken and Vegetable Soup

- Snack: Almond Butter and Banana Rice Cakes

- Dinner: Baked Salmon with Dill Sauce and Roasted Brussels Sprouts

Day 18:

- Breakfast: Overnight Oats with Chia Seeds

- Snack: Apple Slices with Peanut Butter

- Lunch: Thai Beef Salad

- Snack: Hard-Boiled Eggs

- Dinner: Turkey and Veggie Meatballs with Zucchini Noodles

Day 19:

- Breakfast: Breakfast Egg Muffins

- Snack: Berry Frozen Yogurt Bites

- Lunch: Lentil Soup with Whole Grain Bread

- Snack: Greek Yogurt Parfait with Berries

- Dinner: Chicken Stir-Fry with Veggies

Day 20:

- Breakfast: Dark Chocolate Avocado Mousse

- Snack: Mixed Nuts

- Lunch: Grilled Chicken Caesar Salad

- Snack: Veggie Sticks with Hummus

- Dinner: Chicken and Broccoli Casserole

Day 21:

- Breakfast: Mixed Berry Crisp

- Snack: Cottage Cheese with Pineapple

- Lunch: Mediterranean Quinoa Salad

- Snack: Apple Slices with Peanut Butter

- Dinner: Shrimp and Veggie Stir-Fry

Week 4:

Day 22:

- Breakfast: Spinach and Feta Omelette

- Snack: Greek Yogurt with Honey and Nuts

- Lunch: Caprese Salad

- Snack: Almond Butter and Banana Rice Cakes

- Dinner: Lemon Herb Roast Chicken with Roasted Vegetables

Day 23:

- Breakfast: Greek Yogurt Parfait with Berries

- Snack: Mixed Nuts

- Lunch: Butternut Squash Soup with a Side Salad

- Snack: Turkey and Cheese Roll-Ups

- Dinner: Teriyaki Tofu Stir-Fry

Day 24:

- Breakfast: Avocado Toast with Poached Egg

- Snack: Carrot Sticks with Hummus

- Lunch: Chicken and Vegetable Soup

- Snack: Cottage Cheese with Pineapple

- Dinner: Baked Salmon with Dill Sauce and Steamed Broccoli

Day 25:

- Breakfast: Overnight Oats with Chia Seeds

- Snack: Apple Slices with Peanut Butter

- Lunch: Thai Beef Salad

- Snack: Hard-Boiled Eggs

- Dinner: Turkey and Veggie Meatballs with Zucchini Noodles

Day 26:

- Breakfast: Breakfast Egg Muffins

- Snack: Berry Frozen Yogurt Bites

- Lunch: Grilled Chicken Caesar Salad

- Snack: Greek Yogurt Parfait with Berries

- Dinner: Chicken Stir-Fry with Veggies

Day 27:

- Breakfast: Dark Chocolate Avocado Mousse

- Snack: Mixed Nuts

- Lunch: Caprese Salad

- Snack: Veggie Sticks with Hummus

- Dinner: Chicken and Broccoli Casserole

- Dinner: Garlic Butter Grilled Shrimp with Roasted Asparagus

Day 28:

- Breakfast: Mixed Berry Crisp

- Snack: Almond Butter and Banana Rice Cakes

- Lunch: Lentil Soup with Whole Grain Bread

- Snack: Apple Slices with Peanut Butter

- Dinner: Shrimp and Veggie Stir-Fry

Day 29:

- Breakfast: Spinach and Feta Omelette

- Snack: Greek Yogurt with Honey and Nuts

- Lunch: Mediterranean Quinoa Salad

- Snack: Cottage Cheese with Pineapple

- Dinner: Grilled Chicken Skewers with Peanut Sauce

Day 30:

- Breakfast: Greek Yogurt Parfait with Berries

- Snack: Mixed Nuts

- Lunch: Creamy Tomato Basil Soup with a Side Salad

- Snack: Greek Yogurt with Honey and Nuts